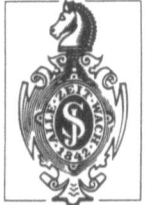

H. Ishikura M. Namiki (Eds.)

Gastric Anisakiasis in Japan

Epidemiology, Diagnosis, Treatment

With 84 Figures, Mostly in Color

Springer-Verlag
Tokyo Berlin Heidelberg New York London Paris

HAJIME ISHIKURA
Honorary Member of the Japanese Society of Clinical Surgery
Director, The Ishikura Hospital
Iwanai, 045 Japan

MASAYOSHI NAMIKI
Professor
The Third Department of Internal Medicine
Asahikawa Medical College
Asahikawa, 078 Japan

ISBN-13: 978-4-431-68292-9   e-ISBN-13: 978-4-431-68290-5
DOI: 10.1007/ 978-4-431-68290-5

© Springer-Verlag Tokyo 1989
Softcover reprint of the hardcover 1st edition 1989

The use of registered names, trademarks, etc. in this publication does not
imply, even in the absence of a specific statement, that such names are
exempt from the relevant protective laws and regulations and therefore free
for general use.

Product liability: The publisher can give no guarantee for information about
drug dosage and application thereof contained in this book. In every individual case the respective user must check its accuracy by consulting other
pharmaceutical literature.

Typesetting: Asco Trade Typesetting, Hong Kong

Preface

The larvae of *Anisakis*, whose adult form lives on sea mammals such as whales, seals, and dolphins, are parasitic upon many species of salt-water fish. When the final host animals eat paratenic hosts, the larvae grow to adulthood in the hosts' stomach. However, when humans eat these infested fish, the larvae die instead, causing a disease called anisakiasis. In 1960, in the Netherlands, van Thiel et al. found a worm in the intestinal wall of a patient who had eaten raw herring and had suffered symptoms of acute abdomen. The impact of this report was tremendous among Japanese parasitologists because of the Japanese habit of eating raw fish. In 1964, the Special Research Group from the Ministry of Education was established to investigate the disease, stimulating progress in the study of anisakiasis.

Three types of worm, *Anisakis simplex* larva (previously known as *Anisakis* larva type I), *Anisakis physeteris* larva (*Anisakis* larva type II), and *Pseudoterranova decipiens* larva type A, are believed to cause anisakiasis. As many as 165 kinds of fish and squid in the seas near Japan are hosts to *Anisakis simplex*, and 9 species are hosts to *Pseudoterranova decipiens* larvae. *Contracaecum* has experimentally been observed to invade the gastrointestinal tract, but no infection by this larva has been reported in humans. A case of infection by *Pseudoterranova decipiens* type B has been described.

In Japan, the name *Terranova decipiens* (Shiraki 1974) has been adopted instead of *Phocanema decipiens* (Mozgovoi 1953). Recently, *Pseudoterranova decipiens* has often been used by parasitologists. The Commonwealth Institute of Helminthology in its publication *Nematode Parasites of Vertebrates* (Hartwich 1974) rejected the term *Pseudoterranova* on the grounds that the initial descriptions of *Pseudoterranova decipiens* by Mozgovoi are incomplete. No systemic nomenclature has been adopted in the present book; the choice of name has been left to the individual authors.

Anisakiasis is categorized into gastric and intestinal forms, each being subdivided into mild and fulminant types. Comprehensive data on the diagnosis and treatment of gastric anisakiasis obtained by fiberscopy, ultrasonography, and double-contrast X-ray study are presented here. Lesions of the gastric mucosa have been examined by fiberscopy. Double-contrast study reveals edema of the gastric mucosa and the body of the worm and is useful for diagnosis. The contrast-dye method shows the worm in localized edematous lesion in the gastric mucosa. The seroimmunological diagnoses, including the use of monoclonal antibodies, which have recently been established, are also described.

Sushi and sashimi have become popular in many parts of the world, and the danger from *Anisakis* is significant. This book is written in the belief that Japanese physicians should make anisakiasis better known in other countries so that the hazards of the disease can be fully recognized.

HAJIME ISHIKURA
MASAYOSHI NAMIKI

Table of Contents

List of Contributors

*Akao, Nobuaki   Lecturer, Department of Parasitology, School of Medicine, Kanazawa University, Kanazawa, 920 Japan

*Asaishi, Kazuaki   Assistant Professor, The First Department of Surgery, Sapporo Medical College and Hospital, Sapporo, 060 Japan

Fujino, Takahiro   Assistant Professor, Department of Parasitology, Faculty of Medicine, Kyushu University, Fukuoka, 812 Japan

Fukuda, Minoru   Director, Fukuda Gastrointestinal Clinic, Miyazaki, 880 Japan

Furusawa, Takeshi   Director, Furusawa Gastrointestinal Hospital, Oita, 879-56 Japan

Hayasaka, Hiroshi   Professor, The First Department of Surgery, Sapporo Medical College and Hospital, Sapporo, 060 Japan

*Hoshihara, Yoshio   Department of Medicine and Physical Therapy, The University of Tokyo, Faculty of Medicine, Tokyo, 113 Japan

*Ishii, Yoichi   Professor, Department of Parasitology, Faculty of Medicine, Kyushu University, Fukuoka, 812 Japan

*Ishikura, Hajime   Honorary Member of Japanese Society of Clinical Surgery; Director, The Ishikura Hospital, Iwanai, 045 Japan

Kikuchi, Kokichi   President and Professor, Department of Pathology, Sapporo Medical College, Sapporo, 060 Japan

*KIKUCHI, YUKO Lecturer, Department of Pathology, Hokkaido University, School of Medicine, Sapporo, 060 Japan

*KUSUHARA, TOSHIYUKI Fukuda Gastrointestinal Clinic, Miyazaki, 880 Japan

MORI, MASAKI The Second Department of Surgery, Faculty of Medicine, Kyushu University, Fukuoka, 812 Japan

*NAGANO, KAZUO Director, Nagano Gastrointestinal Clinic, Hakodate, 040 Japan

NAKAYAMA, TOSHIMICHI Assistant Professor, The Second Department of Surgery, Kurume University, School of Medicine, Kurume, 830 Japan

*NAMIKI, MASAYOSHI Professor, The Third Department of Internal Medicine, Asahikawa Medical College, Asahikawa, 078 Japan

NISHINO, CHISATO Assistant Professor, The First Department of Surgery, Sapporo Medical College and Hospital, Sapporo, 060 Japan

*OOIWA, TOSHIO Director, Ooiwa Gastrointestinal Hospital, Fukuoka, 812 Japan

*OHTAKI, HIDEHO Director, Ohtaki Gastrointestinal Hospital, Fukui, 910 Japan

OHTAKI, REIKO Ohtaki Gastrointestinal Hospital, Fukui, 910 Japan

*SHIBATA, OKIHIKO The Second Department of Surgery, Oita Medical College, Oita, 879-56 Japan

SUGIMACHI, KEIZO Professor, The Second Department of Surgery, Faculty of Medicine, Kyushu University, Fukuoka, 812 Japan

*TAKAHASHI, SYUJI Department of Pathology, Sapporo Medical College, Sapporo, 060 Japan

*TSUJI, MORIYASU Professor, Department of Parasitology, School of Medicine, Hiroshima University, Hiroshima, 734 Japan

UCHIDA, YUZO Assistant Professor, The Second Department of Surgery, Oita Medical College, Oita, 879-56 Japan

WEERASOORIYA, M.V. — Department of Parasitology, Faculty of Medicine, Kyushu University, Fukuoka, 812 Japan

*YANO, MAKOTO — Lecturer, The Second Department of Surgery, Faculty of Medicine, Kurume University, Kurume, 830 Japan

*YAZAKI, YASUYUKI — Lecturer, The Third Department of Internal Medicine, Asahikawa Medical College, Asahikawa, 078 Japan

YOKOMIZO, SEIJI — The Second Department of Surgery, Kurume University, School of Medicine, Kurume, 830 Japan

YOSHIMURA, HIROYUKI — Professor, Department of Parasitology, School of Medicine, Kanazawa University, Kanazawa, 920 Japan

----

*First author

Introduction

H. ISHIKURA

This volume describes several aspects of gastric anisakiasis written by members of advanced study groups in Japan, the country where anisakiasis is most frequent. Unless Japanese change their habit of eating raw fish, this larval contagion will not disappear.

Eating raw fish, such as sushi and sashimi, is also becoming popular in other countries, which will lead to the increased danger of anisakiasis outside Japan. This is a matter of some concern.

Medicaments are usually accompanied by directions on use and details of the side effects. In a similar way, the role of this book is to provide notes concerning the possible dangers associated with the increased consumption of sashimi and sushi.

Larvae of *Anisakis* die when subjected to a temperature of 60°C for 7–10 min and die immediately at 70°C, though this would mean that the fish was no longer raw. They die when frozen at −20°C for 24 h in a refrigerator. This means that from a health point of view, frozen fish should be used for sushi and sashimi, even though this may impair the taste.

In the Netherlands, where anisakiasis was first found, it is statutory for herrings to be frozen prior to consumption and anisakiasis hardly ever occurs as a result of this regulation. Japan has no such regulations as yet, but Japanese doctors should make efforts to establish them.

Certain aspects of anisakiasis are not found in this book. Adult anisakids are parasitic upon the walls of the first stomach of sea mammals and this causes ulcers. Some doctors have suggested the possibility of ulcer formation in the human gastric wall by the larvae.

V. I. Knysh, Chief of the Proctology, Cancer Research Center, USSR Academy of Medical Sciences, Moscow, told me that there is a high rate of gastric cancer among people living around a certain lake in the Soviet Union, probably because they eat freshwater fish, which contain parasites. Desowitz at the Institute of Tropical Medicine and Medical Microbiology, University of Hawaii warns that Japanese should consider the relationship between cancer and anisakiasis because he found that a certain fraction of antigens of *Anisakis* larvae show mutagenic factors and tumor-promoting activity. This needs further study in the future.

Following publication of the present volume, another book "The Advances of

Intestinal Anisakiasis in Japan" is planned. The diagnosis of intestinal anisakiasis is much more difficult than that of the gastric condition. To make a final
diagnosis without surgery is problematic and better diagnostic methods are required. The next book will cover the development of clinical methods such as
X-rays, ultrasonic tomography, intestinal fiberscopy, and the latest findings with
various seroimmunological diagnostic methods. A precise epidemiological and
morphological study of *Anisakis* in the seas around Japan will also be presented
by expert parasitologists. It is to be hoped the next volume, like the present, will
do much to further the knowledge about these parasites and the infections they
cause.

General Survey of *Anisakis* and Anisakiasis in Japan

H. Ishikura

Introduction

A major health hazard associated with the eating of raw fish has been attributed to parasitic infections. Anisakiasis has recently become a leading problem in Japan. Anisakiasis is a disease caused by an infection of *Anisakinae* larvae, which are the visceral larva migrants following an infection by *Anisakis* larvae or related nematodes. It occurs when the live larvae are taken into the human gastrointestinal tract by eating raw, infected fish, in which the larva is in either stage III or IV. It causes pain, and often the pain is so severe that the patient is treated for acute abdominal pain, although the disease is by no means fatal. Anisakiasis was first reported by van Thiel et al. in 1960 in the Netherlands [1], and it has subsequently been reported in the Netherlands [2–4], Japan [5], England [6, 7], the United States [8], as well as other nations. In Japan, as early as 1957, Otsuru et al., who paid particular attention to a study on visceral larva migrants by Beaver [9], raised the possibility that there might also be many cases of visceral larva migrants in Japan, because Japanese eat a great deal of raw fish [10]. The suspicion of Otsuru et al. was followed by findings of patients with anisakiasis by Nishimura in 1963 [5], Asami et al. in 1964 [11], and then Ishikura and Kikuchi in 1967 [12]. The Special Scientific Research Group of the Ministry of Education, founded in 1964 and led by Otsuru, performed nationwide investigations of the disease, contributing much to the understanding of anisakiasis in Japan. Reports on the disease were continuously published in Japan, while Oshima wrote two papers [13, 14], one of which presented detailed Japanese research findings on the disease to the rest of the world [14]. The earlier studies resulted in nationwide recognition of the disease, and there have been more than 1200 papers, in which over 4000 cases of gastric anisakiasis are reported. In the following sections of this chapter, the historical events in the studies of *Anisakinae* and anisakiasis in Japan will be briefly reviewed. For readers convenience, I put the map of Japan, including occurrence of anisakiasis and representative fish that cause most cases of the disease in the area (Fig. 1).

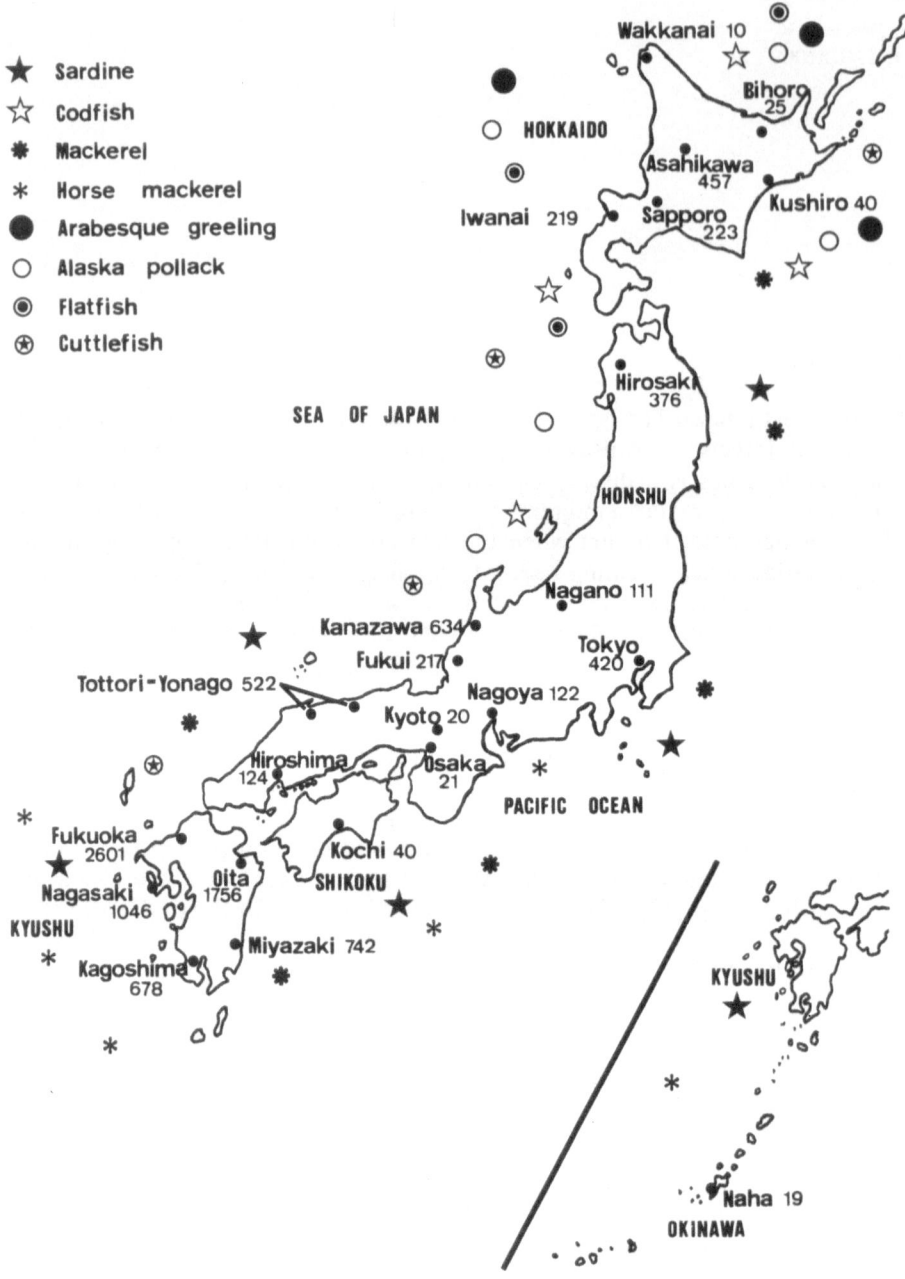

Fig. 1. Occurrence of anisakiasis in major cities in Japan. Numbers represent cases reported from regional hospitals. Species of fish infested by *Anisakis* larvae captured around seas near Japan are also drawn

Studies on *Anisakinae*

Classification of *Anisakinae*

Anisakinae was included among the *Heterocheilidae* in a classification by Yorke and Maplestone [15], but in a more recent classification by Hartwich [59, 60], *Anisakinae* was not included in the *Heterocheilidae* but among the *Anisakidae* (Table 1), because *Heterocheilidae,* which includes only one genus, *Hetero-cheilus,* is different from *Anisakidae* worms in many respects.

Classification of the larvae of *Anisakinae* was confusing until Shiraki proposed a classification with illustrations of cross sections of each larva, and this classification now widely accepted [16]. The following are classified among *Anisaki-nae: Anisakis* (types I, II, III, and IV), *Terranova* (types A, B), *Contracaecum* (types A, B), *Raphidascaris sp.,* and *Thynnascaris.* Recently, *Anisakis* larva type I, type II, and *Terranova* larva type A have been called *Anisakis simplex* larva, *Anisakis physeteris* larva, and *Pseudoterranova decipiens* larva, respectively (Table 2). Oshima et al. also demonstrated serial cross sections of *Anisakis* larvae [17]. These studies made it possible to identify larvae in paraffin-embedded sections.

Confusion remains in the classification of adult forms of *Anisakinae.* Eighteen kinds of adult forms of *Anisakis* have been identified with a great deal of overlap [18, 19], but Oshima classified them into three major groups, as shown in Table 2 [7, 14]. The corresponding larvae of *Anisakinae* are also given in Table 2, but controversy continues on the relation between adults and larvae [14–16, 20]. One of the best methods of discovering the relation between the stages appears to be the culturing of larvae and raising them to adults. The culture method, however, was not available until van Banning cultured *Anisakis* type I larvae into *Anisakis simplex* [21]. In Japan, with the help of van Banning, Oshima and his co-workers could confirm Banning's result. The same method of culturing could be applied to each larva.

On the nomenclature of *Anisakis simplex,* a debate existed as to the larva which most frequently caused anisakiasis. Yamaguti described *Anisakis salaris Yamaguchi* in 1935 [22–27], which was very similar to *Anisakis simplex.* Bychowsky et al. stated that *Anisakis simplex* (Rudolphi, 1908 [61, 62]) was the same as *Anisakis salaris* [28], but Ono regarded *Anisakis simplex* as being the same as *Anisakis dussumierii,* not *Anisakis salaris* [63]. Yamaguti's description was slightly incomplete for a thorough comparison of the characteristics of *Ani-sakis salaris* with those of *Anisakis simplex* and for claiming priority of nomenclature. Therefore, the name *Anisakis salaris* is now disregarded by most investigators. Oshima stated that the confusion was partly due to the fact that identification of the larvae preceded that of the adults with no correlation being made between the two [21].

Life Cycle of *Anisakinae*

Most of the events in the life cycle of *Anisakinae* were described by Kagei [29–32]. In his earlier studies, he described the life cycle as follows. After the eggs contained in the feces of dolphins and other animals, which are the hosts of the

Table 1. *Anisakis* in two different classification systems

	Yorke and Maplestone (1926)	Hartwich (1974)
Phylum	*Nemathelminthes*	*Nemathelminthes*
Class	*Nematoda*	*Nematoda*
Subclass		*Secernentia*
Order	*Eundenatoda*	*Ascaridia*
Superfamily	*Ascaroidea*	*Ascaridoidea*
Family	*Heterocheilidae*	*Anisakidae*
Subfamily	*Anisakinae*	*Anisakinae*
Tribe		*Anisakinea*
Genus	*Anisakis*	*Anisakis*

Table 2. Classification of *Anisakinae*

Adult form	Larval form
Anisakis simplex (Rudolphi, 1908) (with ten synonyms)	*Anisakis* larva type I
Anisakis typica (Diesing, 1860) (with one synonym)	?
Anisakis physeteris (Baylis, 1923) (with three synonyms)	*Anisakis* larva type II
?	*Anisakis* larva type III, IV
Pseudoterranova decipiens	*Terranova* larva type A
?	*Terranova* larva type B
Contracaecum osculatum	*Contracaecum* larva type A
?	*Contracaecum* larva type B, C, D
Raphidascaris sp.	*Raphidascaris* larva type A
Thynnascaris	?

adult worms, are released into the sea, they become the first-stage larvae. Subsequently, the eggs are consumed by tiny crustaceans, such as *Euphausia* or *Thysanoessa* (the first intermediate host), and then become the second- and third-stage larvae. In fish (the second intermediate host) that consume the crustaceans, the larvae become the third and fourth stage. The larvae are then consumed by humans and anisakiasis results. This view, according to which there are significant differences in morphological as well as funcional stages between the forms in the first and second intermediate hosts, was later corrected by Kagei and Kagei et al. [30, 33]. Except for a slight difference in length, there are actually no significant differences between the two forms. Eating infected *Euphausia* or *Thysanoessa,* as well as infected fish, can cause anisakiasis. This version has been widely accepted [34, 35], and fish thus should be regarded as paratenic hosts rather than second intermediate hosts.

Larvae found in patients with anisakiasis in Japan have been in either the third or fourth stage, the latter being a rare finding [36, 37], and no adult worms have been found in the human gastrointestinal tract. Recently, Kliks reported that an adult male worm of *Phocanema decipiens* (*Terranova decipiens*) was found in a

Japanese woman with anisakiasis living in Los Angeles [38]. However, in our experience, anisakiasis caused by an adult worm should be regarded as quite exceptional.

Infected Fish

In fish captured in the sea around Japan, the following larvae of *Anisakinae* have been demonstrated thus far: *Anisakis* (types I–IV), *Terranova* (types A, B), and *Contracaecum*. Kagei and other investigators [39–42] reported that *Anisakis* type I larvae were found in 165 kinds of fish, including sharks [42] as well as squid, *Anisakis* type II in 29 kinds of fish as well as two types of squid, *Terranova* type A in nine kinds of fish, and *Terranova* type B in 15 kinds of fish. In contrast, in patients with anisakiasis, larvae of *Anisakis* (types I, II) and *Terranova* (type A) have been identified. Since larvae of *Contracaecum* have been show to infect animals in experimental studies [43], there may be cases of anisakiasis by *Contracaecum* [44]. In addition, a case with anisakiasis probably due to type B *Terranova* larvae has been reported [45]. Although most cases of anisakiasis in Japan were shown to be caused by *Anisakis* larvae type I, in the United States 67% (16/24) of the cases were found to be due to *Terranova* larvae [8]. Recently, an increasing number of anisakiasis cases caused by *Terranova* larvae have also been reported in Japan since Suzuki et al., reported the first case of "terranovasis" [46–49]. As many as 160 cases of anisakiasis caused by *Terranova* larvae were reported by 1981 [49], but the proportion of the cases attributed to *Terranova* larvae among all anisakiasis cases still remains low in Japan.

There is a discrepancy in the significance of the kind of fish on the development of anisakiasis. Sardines for example, a popular fish in Japan, rarely contain the larvae, according to Kagei [19]. However, in Matsue City and on the island of Kyushu, there have been many anisakiasis patients whose disease was attributed to the eating of sardines [50], the ratio being as high as 11% of all cases in Kyushu on the basis of anamnestic interviews with the patients [51, 52]. This discrepancy may be due to a significant difference in the frequency of infected sardines in various areas, to the manner and frequency of eating fish in different areas, or both.

Studies on Anisakiasis

Anisakiasis was first recognized as its intestinal type in both the Netherlands and Japan. Although the first case of anisakiasis in Japan was reported by Nishimura in 1963 [5], the first clue to nationwide recognition of anisakiasis was seen in a study by Ishikura in 1965, who reported 116 cases of a peculiar form of regional enteritis encountered in a small fishing town, Iwanai [53]. The regional enteritis, which was frequently seen in winter, was characterized by edema and bleeding of the terminal ileum and mesentery. Clinically, it mimicked acute appendicitis and was treated as such. Ishikura could find similar cases reported as nonspecific regional enteritis by Shioda [54] and as acute-type Crohn's disease [55]. He correlated the disease with eating raw Alaskan pollack or their eggs, "tarako" [53, 56]. The enteritis showed acute phlegmonous inflammation in the intestinal wall with marked exudative changes accompanied by eosinophilic infiltration [12]. In the histological sections of affected intestines, cross sections of parasites were sometimes seen, but they were misinterpreted as *Ascaris*. However, Yamaguchi, a parasitologist, identified the parasites as *Anisakis* larvae from the illustrations in Ishikura's paper [53]. Thus, the incidence of as many as 116 cases of anisakiasis in a small fishing town helped investigators in other areas to identify the disease, resulting in a nationwide recognition of the disease.

Later, it was revealed that in addition to the intestinal type described above, there was another type of anisakiasis—the gastric type. In earlier studies, statistics showed that the intestinal type prevailed in the northern part of Japan, while the gastric type prevailed in the southern part. Recent studies, however, have indicated that no such difference exists in the distribution of the two types of anisakiasis. In addition, the intestinal type was once believed to be acute, with the gastric type being exclusively chronic, but many acute cases of the gastric type have been recently found. It is probable that a difference in recognition of the disease, as well as a difference in the utilization of gastrointestinal endoscopy between the northern and southern parts of Japan, led the earlier studies to a somewhat misleading conclusion.

Eating raw fish and their eggs together with the recent remarkable advances in endoscopy seem to be the major reasons why there are so many reported cases of anisakiasis in Japan. Namiki et al., who were some of the earliest investigators to apply gastric fibroscopy to patients with gastric disorders, first demonstrated an *Anisakis* larva attached to the gastric wall in 1970 [57]. That was a major step in the endoscopic diagnosis of anisakiasis. Thereafter, much progress has been seen in the diagnosis and treatment of the disease, which will appear in the subsequent chapters written by the authors who have been responsible for these advances. One particularly great advance is the recent success in raising monoclonal antibodies against *Anisakis* by Takahashi et al. [58], which will add to the immunological diagnosis of anisakiasis in terms of further accuracy and reproducibility.

References

1. van Thiel PH, Kuipers FC, Roskam RT (1960) A nematode parasitic to herring causing acute abdominal syndromes in man. Trop Geogr Med 12: 97–113
2. van Thiel PH (1962) Anisakiasis. Parasitology 52 (suppl): 16–17
3. van Thiel PH, Bakker PM (1981) Wormgranulomen in de maag in Nederland en in Japan. Ned T Geneesk 125 (nr.34): 1365–1370
4. Ruitenberg EJ (1970) Anisakiasis-Pathogenesis, serodiagnosis and prevention. PhD thesis, Rijks University, Utrecht
5. Nishimura T (1963) On a certain nematode larva found in the abscess of the mesentery of a man. Transactions of the 19th Branch-Meeting of Parasit, in the West Division of Japanese Society of Parasitology. Nov. 1963, Okayama, Japan, p 27 (in Japanese)
6. Ashby BS, Appleton P, Dawson I (1964) Eosinophilic granuloma of gastrointestinal tract caused by herring parasite, *Eustoma rotundatum*. Br Med J 1: 1141–1145
7. Smith JW, Wootten R (1978) Anisakis and anisakiasis. Advances in parasitology. Academic, London, pp 93–163
8. Desowitz RS (1986) Human and experimental anisakiasis in the United States. Hokkaido J Med Sci 61: 358–371

9. Beaver PC (1952) Chronic eosinophilia due to visceral larva migrans. Pediatrics 9: 7–19
10. Otsuru M, Ishizuki F, Hatsukano T (1957) Regional ileitis caused by invasion of *Ascarids* larva into intestinal wall. Nippon Ijishimpo 1775: 25–38 (in Japanese)
11. Asami K, Watanuki T, Sakai H, Iwano H, Okamoto R (1964) Two cases of stomach granuloma caused by *Anisakis*-like larvae nematodes in Japan. Am J Trop Med Hyg 14: 119–123
12. Ishikura H, Kikuchi Y (1967) Acute regional ileitis (anisakiasis) at Iwanai district in Hokkaido. Recent advances in gastroenterology. The Third World Congress of Gastroenterology, Sept. 1966, Tokyo, vol. 2. pp 444–446
13. Oshima T (1964) Larva migrans. In: Morishita K, Komiya Y, Matsubashi H (eds) Progress of medical parasitology in Japan, vol 4. Meguro Parasitological Museum, Tokyo, pp 517–548 (in Japanese)
14. Oshima T (1972) *Anisakis* and anisakiasis in Japan and adjacent area. In: Morishita K, Komiya Y, Matsubayashi H (eds) Progress of medical parasitology in Japan, vol 4. Meguro Parasitological Museum, Tokyo, pp 301–393
15. Yorke W, Maplestone PA (1926) Nematode parasites of vertebrates, I and II. Blakiston, Philadelphia
16. Shiraki T (1974) Larval nematodes of family *Anisakidae* (nematoda) in the northern sea of Japan as a causative agent of eosinophilic phlegmone or granuloma in the human gastrointestinal tract. Acta Medica et Biologica 22: 57–98
17. Oshima T, Shimazu T, Akahane H (1967) Comparative morphological studies on the cross section figures of *anisakis* larvae. Jpn J Parasitol 16: 289–290 (in Japanese)
18. Mozgovoi AA (1951) *Ascaridata*. In: Skryabin KI, Shikhobalova NP, Mozgovoi AA. Descriptive catalogue of parasitic nematodesl, vol II. Izdat Akad Nauk SSSR, Moscow, pp 405–566 (in Russian)
19. Kagei K (1967) Two parasite infections caused by raw fishes—The epidemiology and prevention. J Jpn Med Technol 16: 85–102 (in Japanese)
20. Koyama T, Kobayashi A, Kumada M, Komiya Y, Kagei N, Ishii T (1969) Morphological and taxonomic studies on *anisakis* larvae found in marine fish and squids. Jpn J Parasitol 18: 466–487 (in Japanese)
21. Oshima T (1978) Reminiscences of studies on anisakiasis. In: Ishikura H (ed) Anisakiasis. Hokkai Times, Sapporo, pp 459–461 (in Japanese)
22. Yamaguti S (1936) Studies on the helminth fauna of Japan: IX. Nematodes of fishes: I. Jpn J Zool 6: 338–386
23. Yamaguti S (1941) Studies on the helminth fauna of Japan: XXXIII. Nematodes of fishes: II. Jpn J Zool 9: 343–396
24. Yamaguti S (1941) Studies on the helminth fauna of Japan: XXXV. Mammalian: II. Jpn J Zool 9: 423–425
25. Yamaguti S (1942) Studies on the helminth fauna of Japan: XLI. Mammalian nematodes: III. Published by author, pp 5–11
26. Yamaguti S (1958) Systema helminthum: III. The nematodes of vertebrates, part I. Interscience, New York, p 584
27. Yamaguti S (1961) Systema helminthum: III. The nematodes of vertebrates, parts 1, 2. Interscience, New York, pp 1–1261
28. Bychowsky BE, Izumova NA (Translated by Sano T) (1980) Fish parasites—Nemathelminthus. Koseisha Koseikaku, Tokyo, pp 490–495 (in Japanese)
29. Kagei N (1968) Infection and prevention—Raw fishes are dangerous. Kagaku Asahi 28: 97–103 (in Japanese)
30. Kagei N (1969). Life cycle of the genus *Anisakis*. Saishin Igaku 24: 289–400 (in Japanese)
31. Kagei N (1974) Survey of *Anisakis* larvae in the marine crustacea. Jpn J Parasitol 23 (suppl): 8 (in Japanese)
32. Kagei N (1983) Zoonoses-Anisakiasis and Terranovasis. In: Hayashi N, Ishii T, Oshio Y, Koyama T, Kondo S (eds) Buneido, Tokyo, pp 245–257 (in Japanese)
33. Kagei N, Oshima T, Kobayashi A, Kumada M, Koyama T, Komiya Y, Takemura A

(1967). Survey of *Anisakis spp* (*Anisakinae*, Nematoda) on marine mammals on the coast of Japan. Jpn J Parasitol 16: 427–435 (in Japanese)

34. Shimazu T (1974) Ecology of *Anisakid*. Fish and *Anisakis*. Koseisha Koseikaku, Tokyo, pp 23–43 (in Japanese)
35. Nishimura T (1977) Larva nematodiasis, especially on anisakiasis. J Hyogo Med College 5: 237–244 (in Japanese)
36. Ishikura H, Kikuchi Y, Hayasaka Y (1967) Pathological and clinical observations on intestinal anisakiasis. Nippon Gekahokan 36: 663–679 (in Japanese)
37. Fujino T, Oiwa T, Ishii Y (1984) Clinical, epidemiological and morphological studies on 150 cases of acute gastric anisakiasis in Fukuoka prefecture. Jpn J Parasitol 33: 73–92 (in Japanese)
38. Kliks MM (1983) Anisakiasis in the western United States: four new case reports from California. Am J Trop Med Hyg 52: 526–532
39. Kagei N (1974) Studies on *Anisakid* nematoda (*Anisakinae*): IV. Survey of *Anisakis* larvae in the marine crustacea. Bull Inst Publ Health 23: 65–71 (in Japanese)
40. Kagei N, Kureha N (1970) List of the larvae of *Anisakis spp* recorded from marine fish and squids caught off the Japan and its offshore islands. Bull Inst Publ Health 19: 76–85 (in Japanese)
41. Kagei N, Sakaguchi Y, Katamine D, Ikeda Y (1970) Studies on *Anisakid* nematoda (*Anisakinae*): II. *Contracaecum sp* (type IV of Yamaguchi) found in marine fish. Bull Inst Publ Health 19: 243–251 (in Japanese)
42. Suzuki T (1982) On anisakiasis observed in Akita prefecture. Jpn J Parasitol 31: 86 (Suppl) (in Japanese)
43. Otsuru M, Shiraki T, Kenmotsu M (1969) On the morphological classification and experimental infection of *Aniskinae* larvae found in marine fish around the northern sea of Japan. Jpn J Parasitol 18: 417 (in Japanese)
44. Suzuki T (1978) *Anisakis* and *Terranova* larvae, and anisakiasis. In: Otsuru M (ed) Clinical parasitology. Nankodo, Tokyo, pp 300–308 (in Japanese)
45. Saito M, Nozaki K, Suzuki S, Ishizaki T (1978) Terranovasis caused by *Terranova* larva type B: a case report. Gastroenterol Endoscopy 20: 61 (in Japanese)
46. Suzuki H, Ohnuma H, Karasawa S, Yasui A (1972) *Terranova*-like larva picked out from the wall of human stomach with an endoscope. Jpn J Parasitol 21: Suppl. 61 (in Japanese)
47. Iwano H, Ishikura H, Hayasaka H (1974) Statistical analysis of anisakiasis in Japan during the last five years. Geka Shinryo 16: 1336–1342 (in Japanese)
48. Ishikura H, Kikuchi Y, Ishikura H (1983) Enteritis acuta caused by *Anisakis* larvae. Stomach and Intestine 18: 393–397 (in Japanese)
49. Koyama T, Araki J, Machida M, Karasawa Y (1982) Current problems on anisakiasis. Modern Media 28: 434–443 (in Japanese)
50. Ishida A (1984) Three intermediate hostfishes of Anisakis larva in Matsue. In: Ishikura H (ed) Anisakiasis. Kosoku Insatsu Center, Sapporo, p 23 (Suppl 5) (in Japanese)
51. Iino H (1984) Anisakiasis in Kyushu. Gastroenterol Endoscopy 26: 2135 (in Japanese)
52. Matsushita F, Sakaguchi K, Arima T, Kamikozuru K, Hanamura F, Shibue T, Yamashita Y, Hashimoto S (1984) Analysis of 326 cases of anisakiasis occurred at northwest Kagoshima. Gastroenterol Endoscopy 26: 2135 (in Japanese)
53. Ishikura H (1965) Enteritis regionalis exsudativa acuta encountered at Iwanai district in Hokkaido, with special references to its pathological entity. Hokkaido J Surg 10: 29–38 (in Japanese)
54. Shioda H (1939) Nonspecific localized enteritis. J Nippon Med College 10: 1–21 (in Japanese)
55. Crohn BB, Yanis H (1958) Regional ileitis. Grune and Stratton, New York
56. Ishikura H, Tanaka M, Goto T, Aizawa M, Kanemoto T, Ogihara I, Kikuchi K, Tsuji Y, Takahashi T (1965) Studies on regional enteritis: I. Epidemiology of 87 cases at Iwanai district in Hokkaido. Geka Chiryo 13: 144–154 (in Japanese)

57. Namiki M, Morooka T, Kawauchi H, Ueda N, Sekiya C, Nakagawa K, Furuta T, Ooguro T (1970) Diagnosis of acute gastric anisakiasis. Stomach and Intestine 5: 1437–1440 (in Japanese)
58. Takahashi S, Sato N, Sato T, Sato T, Takanmi T, Ishikura H, Mukaiya M, Yagihashi A, Tsurushiin M, Hayasaka H, Kikuchi H (1986) Detection of anti-Anisakis larvae antibodies using micro-ELISA method. Igakuno Ayumi 136: 681–682 (in Japanese)
59. Hartwich G (1957) Zur Systematik der Nematoden-Superfamilie Ascaridoidea. Zool Jb (Syst) 85: 321–326
60. Hartwich G (1974) Keys to Genera of the Ascaridoidea. CIH Keys to the Nematode Parasites of Vertebrates. (eds. Anderson C, Chabaud AG, Willmott S) No. 2: 2–5, Commonwealth Institute of Helminthology, Headley Brothers Ltd, London
61. Pippy JHC, Van Banning P (1975) Identification of *Anisakis* larva (1) as *Anisakis simplex* (Rudolphi, 1908, Krabbe, 1878) (Nematoda: Ascaridata) J Fisheries Res Board Canada 32: 29–32
62. Oya Y, Oshima T, Wakai R (1977) Identification of *Anisakis* larva by *in vitro* cultivation. Jpn J Parasitol 26 (suppl): 78 (in Japanese)
63. Ono Y (1975) Parasitic Zoonoses-Anisakiasis and its prevention. Chikusan no Kenkyu 29: 497–500, 605–610 (in Japanese)

A History of Research into Gastric Anisakiasis in Japan

M. NAMIKI

Progress in Research

Progress in research into gastric anisakiasis in Japan has developed more slowly than research into intestinal anisakiasis. Remarkable and rapid progress, however, has been achieved since 1968 when endoscopic examination allowed the observation of *Anisakis* larvae penetrating the gastric wall and removal and direct identification of the worm. Previously, gastric anisakiasis could only be diagnosed when dead worms and/or their cross sections were histopathologically observed inside granulomas with eosinophilic cell infiltration in the resected stomach. Although the presence of granulomas with eosinophilic cell infiltration in the stomach had been known since the 1950s, Asami et al. [1] confirmed the relation between them and the infection of *Anisakis* larvae in 1964. Their work resulted in the establishment by the Ministry of Education of a research group in 1965 concerned with parasitic granulomas, which was headed by Ohtsuru. In addition, many cases of granulomas with eosinophilic cell infiltration caused by *Anisakis* larvae in the stomach have been reported since 1967. However, it roved difficult to confirm gastric anisakiasis by the conventional method of endoscopic biopsy because the granulomas were too small. This was also found to be the case when granulomas were biopsied with the endoscopic incision method for the submucosal tumors using an electric high-frequency wave. Therefore, the most reliable method seemed to involve obtaining large tissue specimens by jumbo-biopsy.

Endoscopic Diagnosis

Since 1968, Namiki et al. [2] have observed Anisakis larvae penetrating the gastric wall after performing endoscopic examinations on patients showing such acute gastric symptoms as epigastric pain, nausea, and vomiting 4–6 h after eating fresh marine products infected with *Anisakis* larvae. The first case we treated by endoscopy was a 19-year-old female, who had severe epigastric pain 5 h after eating raw squid and cod roe, and the pain lasted 4 days. A worm was endoscopically seen penetrating the anterior wall of the middle body of the stomach. The worm was removed endoscopically with biopsy forceps and identified as an

Anisakis simplex larva. The first endoscopic observation of *Anisakis* larvae on 8 May 1968 was so successful that we have been performing endoscopic examinations ever since. At the 19th Hokkaido Meeting of the Japanese Society of Gastroenterological Endoscopy on 28 September 1969, we presented ten cases of gastric anisakiasis, some of which showed acute gastric symptoms. Furuta of Atsukeshi Choritsu Hospital visited the author 2 weeks after the meeting and brought a worm which had been removed endoscopically. The appearance of the worm was different from *Anisakis simplex* larva. It was bigger, longer, and its color was yellowish brown. The worm was identified as *Pseudoterranova decipiens* larva at the Department of Parasitology, Hokkaido University, School of Veterinary Science. Taking this opportunity, the author requested that physicians routinely check for gastric anisakiasis by trying to establish details of the food eaten, performing endoscopic examination more frequently on patients with acute gastric symptoms, and removing and identifying the worm if found. Furuta experienced three more cases of *Pseudoterranova decipiens* larva at Atsukeshi, a fishing port in the eastern part of Hokkaido, and all cases were found after eating raw turbot. Cases in which *Pseudoterranova decipiens* larva had been removed endoscopically with biopsy forceps were reported by Suzuki et al. [3], Nagano et al. [4], and Kagei et al. [5] in 1972 and by Doi [6] in 1973. Of the 35 worms that Doi [6] removed endoscopically from the stomach, ten were *Pseudoterranova decipiens* larvae, indicating that gastric terranovasis was no longer a rare gastric disease; most cases occurred following the consumption of fresh turbot.

Suzuki and Ishikura [7] and Suzuki [8] divided gastric anisakiasis into two types: a mild type that showed almost no symptoms and formed parasitic granulomas and a fulminant type that showed acute and severe symptoms. General practitioners are currently concerned with the latter. The mechanisms involved in causing the gastric pain are thought to be physical irritation brought about by penetration of the worms into the gastric wall as well as allergic reactions. When I happened to encounter and observe endoscopically the first case of fulminant gastric anisakiasis, I had been inspired by Ishikura's vigorous research work on intestinal anisakiasis and was alert to the possibility of finding *Anisakis* larvae in the stomach. There were two major factors that contributed to the progress in finding and diagnosing anisakiasis: one was Ishikura's influences in arousing attention to the disease among doctors in Hokkaido, including myself; the other was the widespread use of endoscopic examination of the upper gastrointestinal tract in patients showing acute gastric symptoms with an aim to detecting acute gastric mucosal lesions (AGML) and acute gastric lesions (AGL). Having found worms in the stomach by endoscopic examination, Namiki et al. [2], noted that it was possible to take X-ray pictures of the stomach showing the *Anisakis* larvae.

Radiographic Diagnosis

The double-contrast method of stomach X-ray, developed by Shirakabe in 1956 and widely used throughout Japan in the 1960s, was found to be useful in diagnosing the disease by showing the worm as various radiolucent images [9–11].

Thus, upon considering the type of X-ray which visualized the worms, we rechecked all X-ray pictures of the stomach taken of patients exhibiting acute gastric symptoms before 1968. We noted that some pictures taken in the 1960s showed radiolucent images that could be diagnosed as worms. Lack of understanding of gastric aniskiasis was undoubtedly the reason why these images had been overlooked.

Our presentation of many cases of gastric anisakiasis at the 58th Congress of the Japanese Society of Gastroenterology held in Tokyo in March 1972 brought about a nationwide concern regarding gastric anisakiasis with acute gastric symptoms. Many who saw for the first time the pictures of the worms penetrating the gastric wall were surprised, prompting questions regarding the geographic incidence of the disease, whether it was limited to Hokkaido, and whether there were any preventive procedures. I replied that the northern part of Japan had many marine products infected with *Anisakis* larvae and those living in Hokkaido, therefore, were vulnerable to the disease, but that the disease could probably be found in any part of Japan given an awareness its existence. I was later shown to be correct. Cases of endoscopic removal of *Anisakis* larvae have been successively reported from various parts of Japan, and presentations and papers concerning gastric anisakiasis have continued to increase in number since then. Recently, Hirota et al. [12] reported a case of gastric anisakiasis that initially showed a vanishing tumor-like appearance in the fornix of the stomach followed by its disappearance 7 days later. Some cases showing a vanishing tumor-like appearance in the stomach suggest that gastric anisakiasis may have been responsible [13–15].

Ultrasonographic Diagnosis

Ultrasonographic examination [16] has recently been introduced into clinical use as a diagnostic tool. Ultrasonography shows diffuse or local thickening of the gastric wall caused by penetration of the worms. In spite of a remarkable thickening of the wall, peristalsis and elasticity of the wall are retained in gastric anisakiasis in contrast to their loss in malignant diseases of the stomach. In addition, the thickening of the wall characteristically disappears about 1 week after removal of the worms. Noninvasive ultrasonographic examination can be applied to patients with severe abdominal pain on whom it would be difficult to perform endoscopic examination. The most reliable method, however, is to observe the worms endoscopically, to remove them with forceps, and identify them parasitologically. This endoscopic procedure is advantageous diagnostically and therapeutically. The dye-contrast method of spreading 0.1% indigo carmine solution in the stomach may also be helpful in finding the worms [17, 18].

Gastric anisakiasis is nowadays found throughout Japan as general practitioners have become more concerned about the disease and many cases have been reported from various parts of the country [19–23]. At the poster session entitled "Parasites and Endoscopy" at the 27th Convention of the Japanese Society of Gastroenterological Endoscopy held at Asahikawa, Hokkaido in 1984, hosted by the author, there were 13 presentations about gastric anisakiasis. Presentations containing reports of more than 100 diagnosed cases were common, and some reported more than 200. More than 10000 cases have been reported so far in Japan. Most of them were caused by *Anisakis simplex* larva and some by *Pseudoterranova decipiens* larva. Parasitological identification of the worm extracted from the stomach is required because cases due to *Anisakis* larva type II [24] and *Terranova* larva type B [25] have also been reported. Since *Anisakis* larva type II is found mostly in fish in the sea around Okinawa, Kanemitsu et al. [26] point out the possibility of the occurrence of gastric anisakiasis due to *Anisakis* larva type II.

Immunological Research

With regard to immunological research on anisakiasis, including gastric anisakiasis, Takahashi, Hayasaka, Ishikura, Kikuchi et al. of Sapporo Medical College, and Suzuki et al. of the Department of Zoology, Niigata University School of Medicine, among others, have been doing remarkable cooperative reseach [27–33]. Methods for immunological diagnosis are also being studied [34, 35]. Further fundamental research is expected to continue, and progress in the diagnostic procedures is expected to be attained. Our understanding of the disease changes according to the progress in the diagnostic methods and changes in background factors which affect the disease. Further progress in research in this area can only be achieved by the efforts of researchers and an increasing awareness of the disease among general practitioners. Recently, questions regarding fulminant gastric anisakiasis have appeared in the Japanese Medical Board Examination, indicating the nationwide concern about this disease.

It is expected that further developments in the research into anisakiasis will be made by the new generation of researchers.

References

1. Asami K, Watanuki T, Sakai H, Imano H, Okamoto R (1964) Two cases of stomach granuloma caused by anisakis-like larvae nematodes in Japan. Am J Trop Med Hyg 14: 119–123
2. Namiki M, Morooka T, Kawauchi H, Ueda N, Sekiya C, Nakagawa K, Furuta T, Oguro T, Kamata H (1970) Diagnosis of acute gastric anisakiasis. Stomach Intestine 5: 1437–1440 (in Japanese)
3. Suzuki H, Ohnuma H, Karasawa Y, Ohbayashi M, Koyama T, Kumada M, Yokogawa M (1972) Terranova (Nematoda: Anisakidae) infection in man: I. Clinical features of five cases of terranova larva infection. Jpn J Parasit 21: 252–256 (in Japanese)
4. Nagano K, Takagi K, Yanagawa I, Oishi K, Kagei N (1973) Acute hetero-cheilidasis of the stomach (due to Terranova decipiens). Stomach Intestine 8: 81–85 (in Japanese)
5. Kagei N, Yamakawa I, Nagano K, Oishi K (1972) A larva of terranova causing acute abdominal syndrome in a woman. Jpn J Parasit 21: 262–265 (in Japanese)
6. Doi K (1973) Clinical aspects of acute heterocheilidasis of the stomach (due to larvae of anisakis and terranova-decipiens)—Especially on its differential diagnosis by X-ray and endoscopy. Stomach Intestine 8: 1513–1518 (in Japanese)
7. Suzuki T, Ishikura H (1974) Pathogenic mechanisms, symptoms and diagnosis of

anisakiasis. Fishes and Anisakis (no. 7 Fisheries scientific series). Japanese Society of Scientific Fisheries. Kohseisha Kohseikaku, Tokyo, pp 58–72 (in Japanese)

8. Suzuki T (1978) Anisakis and Terranova larva, and Anisakiasis. In: Otsuru M (ed) Clinical parasitology. Nankodo, Tokyo, pp 300–308 (in Japanese)

9. Kawauchi H, Namiki M, Morooka T, Nakagawa K, Oguro T (1973) Gastric anisakiasis presenting acute gastrointestinal symptoms—with special references to the endoscopic and roentgenographic findings of anisakis larva penetrating into the wall of the human stomach and to its clinical features. Stomach Intestine 8: 31–38 (in Japanese)

10. Nakata H, Takeda K, Nakayama T (1980) Radiological diagnosis of acute gastric anisakiasis. Radiology 135: 49–53

11. Sugimachi K, Inokuchi K, Oiwa T, Fujino T, Ishii Y (1985) Acute gastric anisakiasis—analysis of 178 cases. JAMA 253: 1012–1013

12. Hirota K, Uchida Y, Hatano Y, Yasutake R, Okazaki Y, Takemoto T, Fujii Y, Iwata T (1986) A case of gastric anisakiasis taking the course of vanishing tumor of the stomach. Gastroenterol Endosc 28: 780–794 (in Japanese)

13. Yamasaki M (1976) Vanishing tumor of the stomach? Jpn J Clin Radiol 21: 47–54 (in Japanese)

14. Muraoka H, Suzuki S, Okuaki K, Kimura K (1984) A case of "Vanishing tumor of the stomach" due to parasitosis. Gastroenterol Endosc 26: 1719–1724 (in Japanese)

15. Mikami Y (1983) The submucosal tumor due to anisakis larva at the fornix of the stomach. Shimane Med 6: 871–877 (in Japanese)

16. Sakai T, Arima N, Sakemi Y, Majima Y, Toyonaga A, Tanikawa H (1986) Ultrasonographic evaluation of gastric anisakiasis. Jpn J Clin Radiol 31: 949–952 (in Japanese)

17. Hasegawa N, Yoshida S, Yamaguchi H, Tajiri H, Saito O, Hijikata A, Ibe A, Egawa K, Nojiri O, Yoshimori M, Oguro Y, Itabashi M, Hirota T (1984) Usefulness of the simple contrast techinic in endoscopic diagnosis of neoplastic lesions in the stomach. Prog Digest Endosc 25: 113–117 (in Japanese)

18. Hoshihara Y, Yamamoto T, Koyama M, Kawahara H, Kawaguchi Y, Watanabe K (1984) A case of gastric anisakiasis without acute gastrointestinal symptoms, unexpectedly found by contrast dye-method on the endoscopic examination. Prog Digest Endosc 25: 223–225 (in Japanese)

19. Ishikura H (1984) Anisakiasis. Supplement No. 5 ('82–'83). In: Ishikura H (ed) Ishikura hospital. Iwanai, p 7 (in Japanese)

20. Iino H (1984) Anisakiasis in Kyushu. Gastroenterol Endosc 26: 2135 (in Japanese)

21. Matsushita F, Sakaguchi K, Arima T, Kamikozuru K, Nagai T, Shibue T, Yamashita Y, Hashimoto S (1984) Analysis of 326 cases of anisakiasis occurred at northwest Kagoshima. Gastroenterol Endosc 26: 2135 (In Japanese)

22. Fujino T, Oiwa T, Ishii Y (1984) Clinical, epidemiological and morphological studies on 150 case of acute gastric anisakiasis in Fukuoka prefecture. Jpn J Parasitol 33: 73–92 (in Japanese)

23. Omachi K, Omachi T, Maruyama Y (1985) Anisakiasis of gastrointestinal tract in Nagano prefecture. Shinshu Med J 33: 42–56 (in Japanese)

24. Kagei N, Sano M, Takahashi Y, Tamura Y, Sakamoto M (1978) A case of acute abdominal symptome caused by anisakis type-2 larva. Jpn J Parasitol 27: 427–431 (in Japanese)

25. Saito M, Nozaki K, Suzuki S, Ishizaki T (1978) Terranovasis caused by terranova larva type B; a case report. Gastroenterol Endosc 20: 61 (in Japanese)

26. Kanemitsu K, Takara M, Torigoe Y, Satoh Y (1984) A case of anisakiasis in Okinawa. Saishin Igaku 39: 138–141 (in Japanese)

27. Ishikura H (1978) Anisakiasis. Hokkai Times, Sapporo (in Japanese)

28. Nishino C (1977) Epidemiological studies on anisakiasis. Sapporo Med J 46: 73–88 (in Japanese)

29. Suzuki T, Shiraki T, Otsuru M (1969) Studies on the immunological diagnosis of

anisakiasis: II. Isolation and purification of anisakis antigen. Jpn J Parasitol 18: 232–240 (in Japanese)

30. Suzuki T, Otsuru M, Ishikura H (1970) Studies on the immunological diagnosis of anisakiasis: III. Intradermal test with purified antigen. Jpn J Parasitol 19: 1–9 (in Japanese)

31. Suzuki T, Ishida K, Asaishi K, Nishino C (1976) Studies on the immunological diagnosis: VI. Analysis of criteria on intradermal and indirect hemagglutination tests by means of radioimmunoassay. Jpn J Parasitol 25: 17–23 (in Japanese)

32. Takahashi S, Sato N, Sato T, Takami T, Mukaiya M, Yagihashi A, Tsurushiin M, Hayasaka H, Kikuchi K (1986) Detection of antianisakis larva antibodies using micro ELISA method. Igakuno Ayumi 136: 681–682 (in Japanese)

33. Takahashi S, Hayasaka H, Ishikura H, Koshida H, Kikuchi K (1985) Attempts to generate monoclonal antibodies against anisakis larvae. Anisakis, supplement No. 6 ('84–'85). In: Ishikura H (ed) Ishikura hospital, Iwanai, 7 (in Japanese)

34. Yokoya H, Ohe K, Miyoshi A, Hidaka T, Murakami Y, Tsuji M (1980) A study on the diagnosis of three cases of anisakiasis by means of immunoserological techniques. Stomach Intestine 15: 1329–1335 (in Japanese)

35. Tachibana M, Yamamoto Y (1986) Serum anti-anisakis IgE antibody in patients with acute gastric anisakiasis. Jpn J Gastroenterol 83: 2132–2138 (in Japanese)

Morphology of Anisakine Larvae

Y. Ishii, T. Fujino, and M. V. Weerasooriya

At least four species of larval anisakine nematodes can cause human anisakiasis. They include *Anisakis simplex* (Rudolphi, 1809) (*Anisakis* type I), *Anisakis* type II, *Pseudoterranova* (=*Phocanema*) *decipiens* (Krabbe, 1878) (*Terranova* type A), and *Contracaecum sp*. Of these, *A. simplex* and *P. decipiens* are the most common and important anisakids with regard to human infection in Japan as well as some other countries [1]. The larvae of *Anisakis* type II, which penetrate the stomach wall, are regarded as another important pathogen [2]. There is also a report that larvae of *Contracaecum osculatum* (Rudolphi, 1802) found in eosinophilic granulomas of the intestine may be a cause of human anisakiasis in Germany [3]. Since the early taxonomic work of Baylis [4] and Yorke and Maplestone [5], some confusion has existed in the classification of anisakine nematodes, although revised classifications have been proposed by Punt [6], Johnston and Mawson [7], Hartwich [8], Yamaguti [9], Berland [10], and Davey [11]. Recently, Gibson [12] reviewed the systematics of ascaridoid nematodes and commented on the current taxonomic problems; he noted: "*Pseudoterranova* must be recognized as the oldest available name with *Phocanema* as a synonym." He also pointed out that the criteria for distinguishing *Phocanema* and *Pseudoterranova* from *Terranova* are weak and no longer valid. In recent Japanese literature, "*Terranova sp*. larva type A" has been used for *Pseudoterranova decipiens*.

Many studies on the general morphology of anisakine larvae have accumulated, including work by Koyama et al. [13], Shiraki [14], Gibson [15], Oshima [16], and Myers [17]. The external morphological features which help identify the species are differences in the body size, shape, and color and the presence or absence of a mucron at the posterior end. Morphological differences are also found in the internal structures and include the length and shape of the esophagus and ventriculus, the presence or absence of an intestinal cecum, the shape and number of intestinal and excretory cells, the number of somatic muscle cells, and the shape of the lateral cords [14, 16, 18, 19]. These features are especially important in identifying species histopathologically. Recent work using scanning electron microscopy (SEM) has provided a better understanding of the fine morphology of anisakids [20–24].

The third-stage larvae of anisakids from fish molt occasionally to the fourth stage and are ingested by animals and humans. In *A. simplex* and *P. decipiens*, the external as well as the internal morphology change remarkably during molting [15, 23–30].

This chapter deals with the morphological features of the third- and fourth-stage larvae of *A. simplex* and *P. decipiens*, which commonly cause human gastric anisakiasis.

Anisakis simplex (Rudolphi, 1809)

Third-Stage Larvae

This species is most commonly found in various kinds of fish and squid in Japan. The third-stage larvae, threadlike and round in cross section, tend to be longer in northern (average 28.6 mm; 25.2–34.0 mm) [13] than in southern Japan (average 17.0 mm; 12.6–25.1 mm) [31]. According to Oishi et al. [32], the larvae are usually encapsulated within the viscera of fish.

In the anterior end of the larvae, the straight and slender esophagus is followed posteriorly by a thicker ventriculus, which is opaque in transmitted light. The ventriculus forms an oblique junction at the posterior end with the intestine. This morphological feature is diagnostic for larvae of this species.

Observations by SEM have elucidated a number of important surface features [20, 22–24]. The larvae have three low lip bulges at the anterior end, one dorsal and two ventral, which surround the triangular opening of the mouth (Fig. 2). Each subventral lip bulge bears one, while the dorsal lip bulge bears two papilla-like structures. A triangular boring tooth is situated ventrally with the dull end directed outward. The excretory pore, positioned between the bases of the subventral lip bulges, appears as a transverse slit. The cuticular surface has shallow, irregularly spaced, noncontinuous transverse grooves over all the body surface (Fig. 6). Between the transverse grooves are longitudinally running, closely spaced striations formed by fine grooves and ridges. The posterior end of the worm bears a cone-shaped mucron, which varies to some extent in shape (Fig. 10). According to light-microscopic observations by Aihara [20], the mucron has the shape of a spine, pyramid, or knob. He pointed out that the occurrence of each type depends roughly on the species of fish from which the anisakid is removed. In the horse mackerel, the pyramid type is the most common and the knob type the second most common form. An anal duct which leads to a posterior anal pore can be seen under transmitted light at the posterior end of the body. Round anal glands are also located near the posterior end of the intestine. Many of the larvae are encased in a sheath, indicating that molting had already occurred in the fish or human host.

In cross section, the cuticle is thin and uniform in thickness and lacks lateral alae. The lateral cord is composed of a lobular winglike expansion and a narrow stem (Fig. 1A *1–4*). The cord is long in the esophageal region and in posterior sections is pressed to one side. The dorsal and ventral cords are small and inconspicuous throughout the length of the body. The muscle cells are polymyarian type and separated into quadrants by the cords. The muscle cells, 60–90 per quadrant, consist of two parts: a basal fibrillar region and a number of overlying sarcoplasmic processes, which extend into the pseudocoelomic cavity. The excretory cell (renette cell) runs ventrally to the alimentary canal and is attached to the left lateral cord by the left edge of the cell at the margin of the left lateral cord (Fig. 1A *1–3*). The cell begins as a narrow point, is abruptly widened at the level of the esophagus, and then tapers gradually to a fine point. In cross section, the cell is triangular, and extends laterally into a banana-shaped form. A thick-walled tubular excretory canal is seen right to the large, flattened nucleus of the excretory cell. The esophagus is circular in cross section and consists of radially directed muscular fibers, originating from the triradiate lumen and esophageal glandular cells (Fig. 1A *1*). The ventriculus is separated posteriorly into several small sectors by bundles of myofilaments. Some amorphous nuclei can be seen. At the ventriculo-intestinal junction, the intestine occupies a dorsal position. The intestine is composed of 60–80 tall columnar epithelial cells. (Fig. 1A *3–4*). The epithelial cell nuclei are situated near the bases of the cells. The intestinal lumen is triradial of Y-shaped.

Fourth-Stage Larvae

Larvae taken from humans are mostly in the third stage, although some occasionally molt to fourth-stage larvae within 3–5 days after ingestion [15, 23, 29, 33]. The third-stage larvae are also known to molt when they are fed experimentally to rats, rabbits, dogs, and cats [15, 25–28, 34, 35]. After molting, an increase in the head width occurs, although there is no significant increase in the length of the worm [15]. The characteristic features observed under the light microscope of the fourth-stage larvae are: (a) absence of the boring tooth at the anterior end and the mucron at the posterior end; (b) the presence of the three well-defined lips; (c) the appearance of regular transverse striations on the cuticle; (d) the appearance of a pair of small papillae at the cervical area; (e) the presence of a pair of phasmids near the posterior end; (f) the appearance of altered configurations in the ventriculus and intestine; and (g) the development of a reproductive system in female specimens.

   There have been some SEM observations of fourth-stage larvae [20, 23, 24, 36]. The features elucidated under the SEM are as follows. The larvae have three distinct lips (Fig. 3). The dorsal lip is bigger than the two subventral lips. These three lips surround the triangular opening of the mouth cavity. A pair of papillae is located on the dorsal lip and one on each of the subventrals. These papillae double up to form larger (outer labial) and smaller (cephalic) papillae. Two other outer labial papillae are located on each subventral lip as small round elevations. A single dentigerous ridge extends along the median border of each bilobed lip. Each dentigerous ridge has 35–45 single or bifurcate denticles. The denticles on the subventral lip appear broader and shorter than those on the dorsal lip. The cuticle is characterized by transverse grooves, which are regularly spaced and continuous (Fig. 7). Higher magnifications demonstrate that these grooves are formed by two units—a shallow and a deep furrow. Longitudinal fine striations between the transverse grooves appear finely waved. At the posterior end of the body the mucron is absent, and two different features appear: a cone-shaped structure, depressed at the tip and studded with many small spherical elevations (Fig. 11), and three cuticular elevations, the central of which is slightly higher than the other two. There are two phasmids situated symmetri-

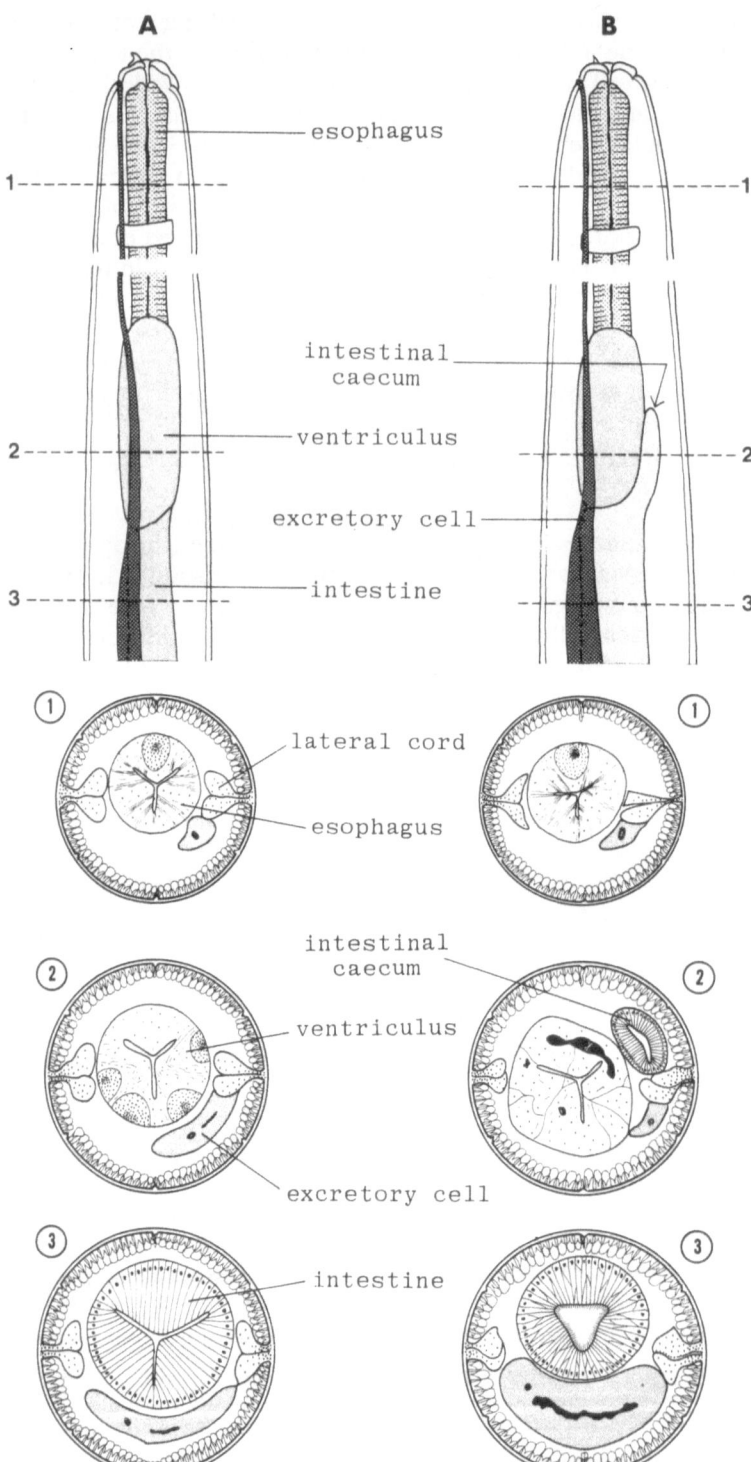

Fig. 1

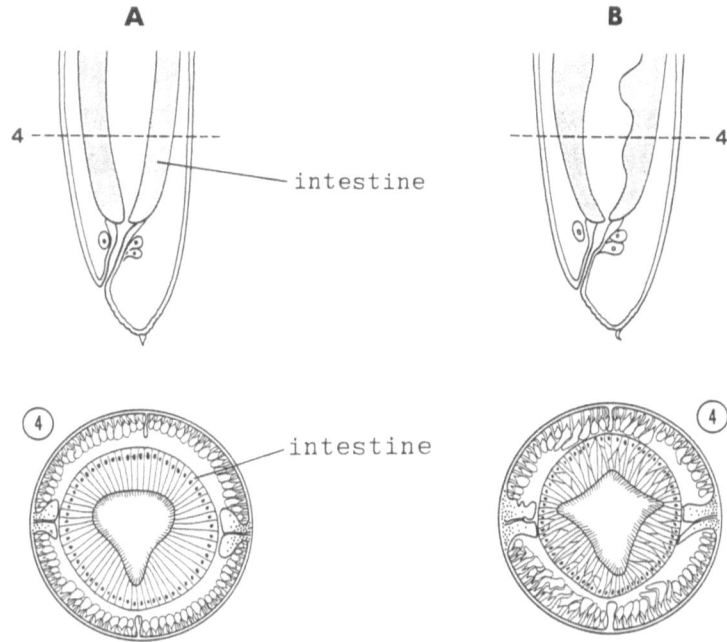

Fig. 1A, B. Diagrammatic representation of the third-stage larvae of **A** *Anisakis simplex* and **B** *Pseudoterranova decipiens*. Level of cross section is indicated by the *broken lines* (*1–4*)

cally, which appear as round elevations surrounded by a distinct groove.

In cross section, the lateral cords are smaller and narrower than those from third-stage larvae; the lateral cords have two distal lobes that are fused into a small curved lobe in fourth-stage larvae. The right lateral cord is broader than the left. The excretory cell appears to be folded basally. It is triangular in cross section at its anterior end and becomes oblong near its posterior end. The cell is attached to the left lateral cord near the anterior end and is detached from it at the level of the ventriculus. The ventriculus is roughly quadrate in cross section, with a ragged outer surface. The lumen of the ventriculus is seen dorsally as a wide transverse slit whose outline is uneven. This slit is larger posteriorly, leading to the round intestinal lumen. The intestine is diamond-shaped and somewhat wavy in outline. The epithelial cells are separated into groups by the irregularly subdivided deep lumen. Each group of cells is roughly triangular or semicircular, the central cells being taller than the lateral ones. The nuclei are located near the bases of the cells. The female larvae have a developing reproductive organ in the middle of the body, which consists of a short vagina and separated uteri [15, 23]. The vulva is not opened to the outside. The development of a male system has not been observed [15].

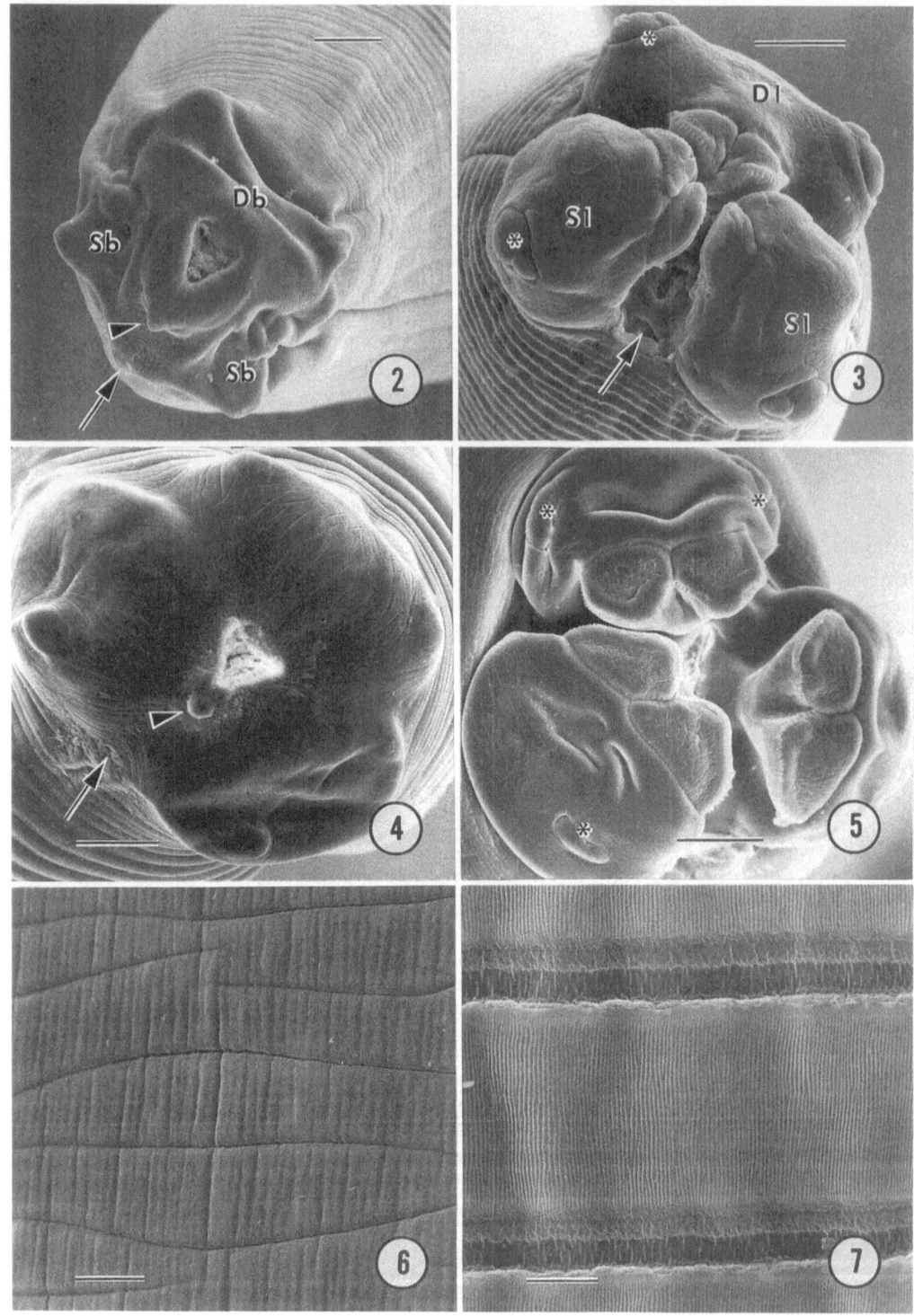

Pseudoterranova decipiens (Krabbe, 1878)

Third-Stage Larvae

This species is commonly found in muscles of fish captured in northern Japan. It is rarely encapsulated. This worm is apparently larger and thicker than *A. simplex*, measuring on average 34.1 mm in length (29.7–4.0 mm) [37]. It is colored brown or occasionally reddish or yellowish. In live worms, the whitish ventriculus, partly covered by the intestinal cecum at its posterior edge, can be seen through the body wall [32, 38].

SEM studies revealed the following detailed morphology of this species [22, 24]. The third-stage larva is similar to that of *A. simplex*, except that the lip bulges are much more prominent and well demarcated (Fig. 4). The boring tooth, situated ventral to the triangular mouth opening, is directed outward. The position and shape of the excretory pore is similar to that of *A. simplex*. The bases of the lip bulges exhibit papilla-like structures, but higher magnifications reveal them to be swellings of the cuticular bases. The cuticular pattern of the body is similar to that of *A. simplex*, and the transverse grooves are composed of two different types: one is narrow and the other broader with a banded appearance (Fig. 8). Irregular shallow longitudinal ridges are seen between the transverse grooves. At the posterior end of the body is a small mucron, which is longer and more slender than in *A. simplex*; it is often curved in the distal half (Fig. 12).

Cross sections of *P. decipiens* are much larger than those of *A. simplex*. The lateral cord consists of two cells, which are expanded broadly into a butterfly-like shape with a broad stem (Fig. 1B*1–4*). Unlike *A. simplex*, the distal expansion is not divided. The muscle cells are similar to those of *A. simplex* and the number about 70 per quadrant. The excretory cell runs ventral to the alimentary

---

Fig. 2. *Anisakis simplex*, third-stage larva, anterior end. *Arrowhead* indicates a boring tooth. *Arrow* shows the excretory pore. *Db* dorsal lip bulge, *Sb* subventral lip bulge. SEM, *scale bar* 30 μm

Fig. 3. *Anisakis simplex*, fourth-stage larva, anterior end, showing well-defined lips with the dentigerous ridges. *Arrow* indicates the excretory pore. *Asterisk* shows a doubled papilla. *Dl* dorsal lip, *Sl* subventral lip. SEM, *scale bar* 30 μm

Fig. 4. *Pseudoterranova decipiens*, third-stage larva, anterior end. *Arrowhead* indicates a boring tooth. *Arrow* shows the excretory pore. SEM, *scale bar* 30 μm

Fig. 5. *Pseudoterranova decipiens*, fourth-stage larva, anterior end, showing well-defined lips with the W-shaped dentigerous ridges. *Asterisk* indicates a papilla. SEM, *scale bar* 30 μm

Fig. 6. *Anisakis simplex*, third stage larva, mid-cuticle, showing irregular transverse grooves. SEM, *scale bar* 5 μm

Fig. 7. *Anisakis simplex*, fourth-stage larva, mid-cuticle, showing regular transverse grooves and fine linear longitudinal ridges between the grooves. SEM, *scale bar* 5 μm

canal, being attached to the left lateral cord (Fig. 1B*1–3*). The cell is oblong or oviform at the level of the esophagus. In the middle of the cell, there is an excretory canal with a thick wall anteriorly. The canal is eccentrically located posteriorly. At the level of the ventriculus, the excretory cell is narrow and then expands to a thick banana-shaped form at the level of the upper intestine. The ventriculus is quadrate and has a spongy texture, occupying the majority of the body cavity in cross section (Fig. 1B2). The intestinal cecum reaches the level of the middle of the ventriculus and is attached to the lateral cord by the right edge (Fig. 1B2). The cecum is oblong and is composed of single columnar epithelium, the cells being about 50 in number. The intestinal epithelium has about 100 tall columnar cells (Fig. 1B*3–4*).

Oshima [16] pointed out some characteristic features, which help to distinguish this species from *A. simplex*: more than 100 intestinal cells, butterfly-like lateral cords, and the presence of an intestinal cecum.

Fourth-Stage Larvae

According to a few reports, the third-stage larvae molt to the fourth when ingested by humans or animals [24, 30, 39]. The molting occurs 3 days after infection in rats [24]. The fourth-stage larvae, as seen in *A. simplex*, show some characteristic morphological features which differ markedly from those of the third-stage larvae. Detailed observations have been made using SEM [24].

At the anterior end are prominent lips, equal in size and shape (Fig. 5). The bilobed medial region of the lips appears much more prominent and larger than in *A. simplex*. The dentigerous ridges surmount the medial borders of the lips and exhibit a well-defined W-shape. Each dentigerous ridge consists of about 45–50 bifurcate denticles and a few denticles with a single point. The denticles in all three lips are much longer and thinner than those of *A. simplex*. Four papillae are observed: two lie on the dorsal lip and one at the base of each of the subventral lips. These papillae are oval, flat, and well demarcated by a shallow groove.

Fig. 8. *Pseudoterranova decipiens*, third-stage larva, mid-cuticle, showing two different types of grooves. SEM, *scale bar 5 μm*

Fig. 9. *Pseudoterranova decipiens*, fourth-stage larva, mid-cuticle, showing clear transverse grooves, which are increased in number. SEM, *scale bar 5 μm*

Fig. 10. *Anisakis simplex*, third-stage larva, posterior end, with a curved mucron. SEM, *scale bar 10 μm*

Fig. 11. *Anisakis simplex*, fourth-stage larva, posterior end, having a cone-shaped structure with a depressed tip and studded spherical elevations. SEM, *scale bar 10 μm*

Fig. 12. *Pseudoterranova decipiens*, third-stage larva, posterior end, with a spinelike mucron. SEM, *scale bar 10 μm*

Fig. 13. *Pseudoterranova decipiens*, fourth-stage larva, posterior end, with a knoblike process and small spherical elevations. *Arrowhead* indicates a phasmid. SEM, *scale bar 10 μm*

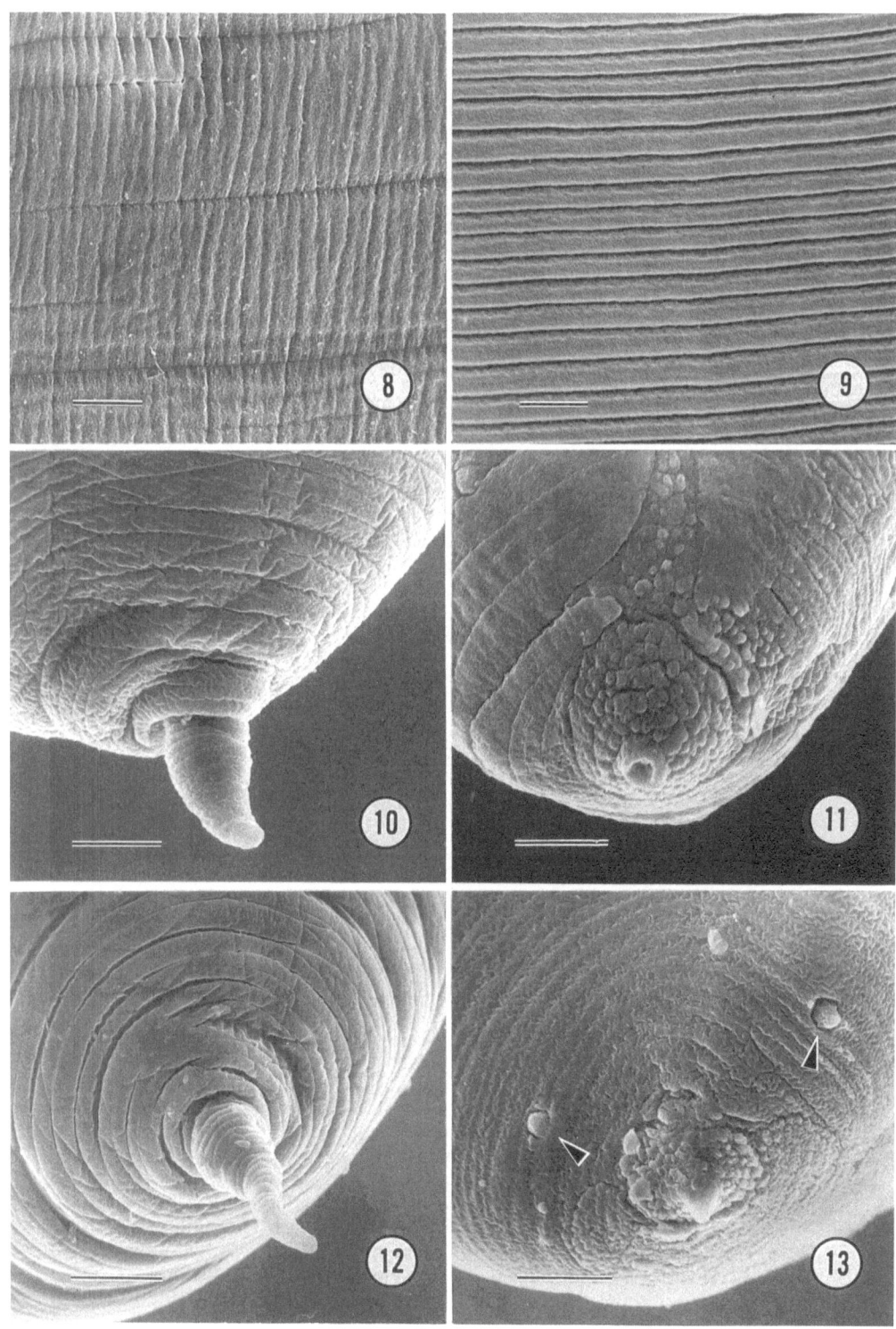

A slight depression in the middle shows them to be double structures. Many more transverse grooves are located in the cuticle than in the third stage (Fig. 9). Each groove is broader, regularly spaced, and continuous. Longitudinal striae are irregular and ill-defined by an anterior wrinkled edge. At the posterior end, a knoblike process surrounded by a large number of spherical elevations is seen (Fig. 13). Two phasmids are seen bilaterally as flat, round, single structures. McClelland [30] experimentally infected *P. decipiens* larvae in seals and obtained fourth-stage larvae 48 h to 9 days postinfection. He noted: "In ensheathed and recently molted L4 (fourth stage larvae), there were genital primordia similar to those in the L3 (third stage larvae). In advanced L4 females, there were rudimentary vagina, uterus, and ovaries; in males, a rudimentary vas deferens and spicule primordia."

References

1. Koyama T, Araki J, Machida M, Karasawa Y (1982) Current problems on anisakiasis. Modern Media 28: 434–443 (in Japanese)
2. Kagei N, Sano M, Takahashi Y, Tamura Y, Sakamoto M (1978) A case of acute abdominal syndrome caused by *Anisakis* type-II larva. Jpn J Parasitol 27: 427–431
3. Schaum E, Müller W (1967) Die Heterocheilidiasis. Eine Infektion des Menschen mit Larven von Fisch-Ascariden. Dtsch Med Wochenschr 92, 2230–2233
4. Baylis HA (1920) On the classification of the Ascaridae: I. The systematic value of certain characters of the alimentary canal. Parasitology 12: 253–264
5. Yorke W, Maplestone PA (1925) The nematode parasites of vertebrates. Blakiston, Philadelphia, pp 1–536
6. Punt A (1941) Recherches sur quelques nématodes parasites de poissons de la Mer du Nord. Mém Mus Roy Hist Nat Belgique 98: 1–110
7. Johnston TH, Mawson PM (1945) Parasitic nematodes. In Rep. B. A. N. Z. Antarctic Res. Exped., 1919–1931, Ser. B. vol. 5, pp 73–159
8. Hartwich G (1957) Zur Zystematik der Nematoden-Superfamilie Ascaridoidea. Zool Jb (Syst.) 85: 211–252
9. Yamaguti S (1961) Systema Helminthum: III. The nematodes of vertebrates, parts 1, 2. Interscience, New York, pp 1–1261
10. Berland B (1961) Nematodes from some Norwegian marine fishes. Sarsia 2: 1–50
11. Davey JT (1971) A revision of the genus *Anisakis* Dujardin, 1845 (Nematoda: Ascaridata). J Helminthol 45: 51–72
12. Gibson DI (1983) The systematics of ascaridoid nematodes—a current assessment. In: Stone AF, Platt HM, Khalil LF (eds) Concepts in nematode systematics, vol. 22. Academic, London, pp 321–338
13. Koyama T, Kobayashi A, Kumada M, Komiya Y, Oshima T, Kagei N, Ishii T, Machida M (1969) Morphological and taxonomical studies on Anisakidae larvae found in marine fishes and squids. Jpn J Parasitol 18: 466–487 (in Japanese)
14. Shiraki T (1969) Histopathological diagnosis of the larva migrans in the digestive tract. Saishin Igaku 24: 378–389 (in Japanese)
15. Gibson DI (1970) Aspects of the development of 'herring worm' (*Anisakis* sp. larva) in experimentally infected rats. Nytt Mag Zool 18: 175–187
16. Oshima T (1972) *Anisakis* and anisakiasis in Japan and adjacent area. In: Morishita K, Komiya Y, Matsubayashi H, (eds) Progress of Medical Parasitology in Japan, vol. 4. Meguro Parasitological Museum, Tokyo, pp 301–393
17. Myers BJ (1975) The nematodes that cause anisakiasis. J Milk Food Technol 38: 774–782

18. Oshima T, Shimazu T, Akahane H (1967) Comparative morphological studies of the cross section figures of anisakid larvae. Jpn J Parasitol 16: 289–290 (in Japanese)
19. Koyama T, Kobayashi A, Kumada M, Omibuchi Y, Oshima T, Kagei N, Ishii T, Machida M (1969) Histological study on Anisakidae larvae found in marine fishes and squids. Jpn J Parasitol 18: 353–354 (in Japanese)
20. Aihara Y (1973) Morphological studies on *Anisakis* larvae type I. J Osaka City Med Center 22: 197–235, Pls 1–5 (in Japanese)
21. Aji T, Tongu Y, Harada M, Itano K, Inatomi S, Suguri S (1981) Fine morphology of head part and mucron in Anisakidae larva. Jpn J Parasitol 30: [Suppl] 109 (in Japanese)
22. Valter ED, Popova TI, Valovaya MA (1982) Scanning electron microscope study of four species of anisakid larvae (Nematoda: Anisakidae). Helminthologia 19: 195–209
23. Fujino T, Ooiwa T, Ishii Y (1984) Clinical, epidemiological and morphological studies on 150 cases of acute gastric anisakiasis in Fukuoka Prefecture. Jpn J Parasitol 33: 73–92 (in Japanese)
24. Weerasooriya MV, Fujino T, Ishii Y, Kagei N (1986) The value of external morphology in the identification of larval anisakid nematodes: a scanning electron microscope study. Z Parasitenkd 72: 765–778
25. Myers BJ (1963) The migration of *Anisakis*-type larvae in experimental animals. Can J Zool 41: 147–148
26. Usutani N (1966) Histological studies on experimental animals administered with *Anisakis*-like larvae from marine fish (Studies on larva migrans, Part 3). Shikoku Acta Medica 22: 486–503 (in Japanese)
27. Koyanagi T (1967) Experimental studies on the visceral migrans of gastrointestinal walls due to *Anisakis* larvae. Jpn J Parasitol 16: 470–493 (in Japanese)
28. Young PC, Lowe D (1969) Larval nematodes from fish of the subfamily Anisakinae and gastro-intestinal lesions in mammals. J Comp Pathol 79: 301–313
29. Akasaka Y, Matsuno K, Yoshida Y, Arizono N, Ikai T, Ogino K, Takeuchi S, Yamada M (1977) Endoscopical treatment of gastric anisakiasis with special reference of ecdysis of *Anisakis* type I larva in the human stomach. J Kyoto Pref Univ Med 86: 257–260 (in Japanese)
30. McClelland G (1980) *Phocanema decipiens*: molting in seals. Exp Parasitol 49: 128–136
31. Sakaguchi Y, Katamine D (1971) Survey of anisakid larvae in marine fishes caught from the East China Sea and the South China Sea. Tropical Med 13: 159–169 (in Japanese)
32. Oishi Y, Fukita H, Suzuki M (1974) Characteristic features identifying live anisakid larvae (addition). In: Japanese Society of Fisheries (ed) Fishes and anisakids. Fish Sci ser. 7, Koseisha-koseikaku, Tokyo pp 20–22 (in Japanese)
33. Nishimura T (1969) Ecology of *Anisakis* larvae. Saishin Igaku. 24: 405–412 (in Japanese)
34. Grainger JNR (1959) The identity of the larval nematodes found in the body muscles of the cod (Gadus callarias L.). Parasitology 49: 121–131
35. Asami K, Inoshita Y (1967) Experimental anisakiasis in guinea pigs: factors influencing infection of larvae in the host. Jpn J Parasitol 16: 415–422
36. Ishii Y, Iino H, Kagei N (1972) Scanning electron microscopy of helminths: VI. *Anisakis* larva. Igakuno Ayumi 81: A-283-284 (in Japanese)
37. Koyama T, Kumada M, Suzuki H, Ohnuma H, Karasawa Y, Ohbayashi M, Yokogawa M (1972) *Terranova* (Nematoda: Anisakidae) infection in man: II. Morphological features of *Terranova* sp. larva found in human stomach wall. Jpn J Parasitol 21: 257–261
38. Oishi Y (1973) Arabesque greenling and *Terranova* larvae. Food Industry 16: 75–84 (in Japanese)
39. Lichtenfels JR, Brancato FP (1976) Anisakid larva from the throat of an Alaskan Eskimo. Am J Trop Med Hyg 25: 691–693

Geographical Distribution and Epidemiology

K. Asaishi, C. Nishino, and H. Hayasaka

Introduction

Anisakiasis, which is caused by *Anisakis* larvae, is one of the most important parasitic diseases of the gastrointestinal tract in Japan [1]. The clinical features of anisakiasis are characterized by a number of acute abdominal symptoms. It is characterized microscopically by an eosinophilic inflammation of the surrounding invading larva. In this chapter, epidemiological studies of anisakiasis are described.

Geographic Distribution and Epidemiology

There are no specific regional characteristic, but most cases are reported at medical facilities located near coastal regions [1]. The outbreak of this disease occurs from December to March in the northern region and from February to May in the southern region of Japan. The cause is related to the movement of paratenic host fish. The kinds of paratenic host fish differ in the south and north. The main paratenic host fish are cod and squid in the northern region and mackerel, sardines, horse mackerel, and cuttlefish in the southern region [2]. *Anisakis simplex* mainly live upon the dolphin, which swims about in the Pacific Ocean. *Anisakis simplex* larvae have been mainly recognized in many paratenic host fish in the Sea of Japan. Almost all cases caused by *Terranova* larvae have been reported in the northern region. The adult nematodes may live in the seal or fur seal [1]. The host animal of *Terranova* usually lives in the Sea of Okhotsk and a great many cases of terranovasis have been reported in the northern region [1]. Anisakiasis is caused by the migration of the third-stage larvae to the wall of the human alimentary tract.

   The total number of recorded gastric anisakiasis cases in Japan according to a nationwide statistical survey was 11 232 in 1988 [3]. Ishikura has reviewed the Japanese literature until 1988. He gave a detailed account of anisakiasis at the 35th Congress of Japanese Gastroenterological endoscopy [3]. Fukumoto reported on 222 cases of gastric anisakiasis, which had been diagnosed by endoscopic examination [2]. He recognized 87 cases of *Anisakis simplex* larvae. Yoshimura examined histologically 634 cases of anisakiasis from 1979 to 1983 [2]. He

Table 1. Age and sex distribution of gastric anisakiasis

Age (years)	Male	Female	Total
–9	0	1	1 (0.3%)
10–19	1	8	9 (2.7%)
20–29	40	29	69 (20.7%)
30–39	76	43	119 (35.6%)
40–49	39	31	70 (20.9%)
50–59	27	20	47 (14.1%)
60–69	11	4	15 (4.5%)
70–79	3	0	3 (0.9%)
80–	0	1	1 (0.3%)
Total	197	137	334 (100.0%)

identified parasitologically 76 cases of *Anisakis simplex* larvae and 18 cases of *Pseudoterranova decipiens* larvae. Karasawa reported on 224 cases in Hokkaido, the northernmost island of Japan [2]. Seventy percent of these larvae were recognized as *Anisakis* larvae parasitologically, and 30% of *Pseudoterranova decipiens* larvae.

A nationwide investigation on the incidence of anisakiasis over a period of 5 years from 1973 through 1977 was conducted by means of a questionnaire sent to 851 major medical centers throughout Japan, which were sent in particular to the departments of parasitology, medical zoology, and pathology [4, 5]. The number of cases for all Japan over the 5-year period was 334 cases of gastric anisakiasis [5]. The age and sex distribution of gastric anisakiasis are shown in Table 1. In terms of age, a high rate of incidence was seen mostly between 20 and 50 years, with the highest rate at age 30 (195 patients were male and 139 were female). The youngest patient was a 3-year-old female in whom *Anisakis* larvae were discovered in the vomit; the oldest patient was an 80-year-old female. Adults, particularly males aged 20–40 years, are the most common sufferers because of the frequency of eating raw fish.

Recently, quite a number of cases involving anisakiasis have been reported in Japan and thus it seems reasonable to state that the nematodes found in the human digestive tract are closely linked to the Japanese custom of eating raw fish, such as sashimi and sushi (Table 2). The variety of marine products and the processing of raw fish which cause anisakiasis are shown in Table 2. The number of cases of anisakiasis caused by eating slightly vinegared mackerel has increased recently in the southern compared with the northern region. Processed raw fish, in particular salted roe, has also become a large problem (Table 2). The occupation of patients with gastric anisakiasis showed a wide range in our survey (Table 3).

Random groups of inhabitants living in Hokkaido together with patients with gastric anisakiasis were investigated immunologically using a skin test, by indirect hemagglutination test (IHA), and measurement of serum IgE [6]. Specific antigens against *Anisakis* larvae hemoglobin were used in these experiments. The following subjects were studied: 42 patients with acute gastric anisakiasis, a

Table 2. Variety of marine products causing anisakiasis

Sashimi, sushi	Number
Flatfish	87
Tuna	44
Cod	39
Cuttlefish, squid	33
Greenling	15
Yellowtail	11
Trout	3
Other	41
Processed raw fish	
Vinegared mackerel	79
Salted	
Roe	13
Cod	6
Salmon	3
Dace	1
Other	3
Fermented fish	7
Frozen fish	2

Table 3. Occupation and gastric anisakiasis

Occupation of patient	No. of cases
White-collar worker	85
Housewife	82
Farmer	31
Public servant	22
Laborer	15
Cook, restaurant worker	12
Taxi driver	11
Medical doctor, nurse	6
Store clerk	4
Teacher	3
Policeman	3
Engineer	3
Student	3
Fisherman	3
Unemployed	8
Unknown	43
Total	334

group of 2592 inhabitants ranging in age from 20 to 82 years, 375 high school students 16–18 years old, and 141 children aged 4–5 years (Table 4). All cases of gastric anisakiasis showed a positive reaction to the skin test, and 89.2% showed a positive reaction to IHA. Generally, a tendency to show high levels of serum total IgE was seen and 76.9% revealed the presence of IgE to *Anisakis* larvae. General inhabitants showed 63%, the high school students 29.3%, and the young children 2.1% positive rate. In the IHA test, it was seen that a positive reaction occurred in 36.6% of the inhabitants and 19.5% of high school students (Table 4). No significant difference was seen between the incidence of male and female positive reactions. Likewise, no significant difference was observed in the age levels of general inhabitants. In inhabitants in whom both skin tests and IHA tests were conducted, the four categories were set up and investigated (Table 5). It is believed that types I, II, and III, which show a positive reaction in one or both skin tests or the IHA tests, have antibodies to *Anisakis* larvae. Inhabitants living in areas associated with the fishing industry showed a high positive rate to the skin test and IHA, while inhabitants of farming areas showed a low positive rate in both tests. The difference in these positive rates may be related to the frequency of eating raw fish. The serum total IgE level of the positive group in the skin test was remarkably higher than that of the negative group (Fig. 1). The serum-specific IgE had a high incidence (71.8%) within the skin test-positive group, while a low incidence (4.1%) was seen in the negative group. The patients with anisakiasis were subdivided according to their etiology, i.e., whether the reaction was anaphylactic or the Arthus type: (a) Combined type (reaction to both); (b) anaphylactic reaction type; (c) Arthus reaction type; (d) type showing simple inflammatory reaction to the foreign body.

Table 4. Epidemiological survey in Hokkaido (positive rate)

	Skin test		IHA	
	Percent	No.	Percent	No.
Patients	100	42/42	90.5	38/42
Adults	63.0	1491/2365	36.6	760/2077
High school students	29.3	110/375	19.5	48/246
Young children	2.1	3/141	—	

IHA indirect hemagglutination test

Table 5. Normal subjects divided according to the different antibodies to *Anisakis* larvae

	Cytotropic antibody (IgE)	Serum antibody (mainly IgE)
Type I	(+)	(+)
Type II	(+)	(−)
Type III	(−)	(+)
Type IV	(−)	(−)

Discussion

We would like to point out that gastric anisakiasis may at times account for those gastric diseases usually regarded as acute gastritis, food poisoning, or gastric cramp. It was noted that in the diagnosis of anisakiasis, positive clues may be frequently obtained by anamnesis. Until recently, most cases of gastric anisakiasis were diagnosed by physicians following X-ray or endoscopic examination. A larva penentrating the gastric wall is often evident in a double-contrast radiograph. Using this technique, the *Anisakis* larva appear as a linear translucency of various shape. Fiberscopic examination also reveals the *Anisakis* larva penetrating the gastric wall. With the fiberscope, the larva is observed to be quite transparent and whitish, exhibiting a notable, brisk, winding movement. In most cases, removing the larva with biopsy forceps under direct vision results in the rapid relief of severe epigastric pain. In the diagnosis of acute gastric anisakiasis, gastroendoscopy is highly effective. Anisakiasis is characterized histologically by an eosionophilic phlegmon, abscess, or granuloma formation. In many instances, a migrating larva is found in routine histological sections, but in some cases, the larva is missing, so that as many sections as possible have to be examined to locate the larva when the characteristic tissue reaction of anisakiasis are evident.

It is believed that an allergic reaction plays a role in the etiological mechanism of anisakiasis [6–9]. One premise of the onset of the disease is that the human body has been previously infected by *Anisakis* larvae and is in a sensitized state [7, 8]. We have demonstrated that the etiological mechanism of anisakiasis involves an anaphylactic reaction as well as an Arthus reaction in the alimentary tract [10]. Cell-mediated immune reactions must also be considered in estab-

Fig. 1. Distribution of total IgE
values in each group. A clear difference was seen between skin test-
positive types I and II and the skin
test-negative types III and IV

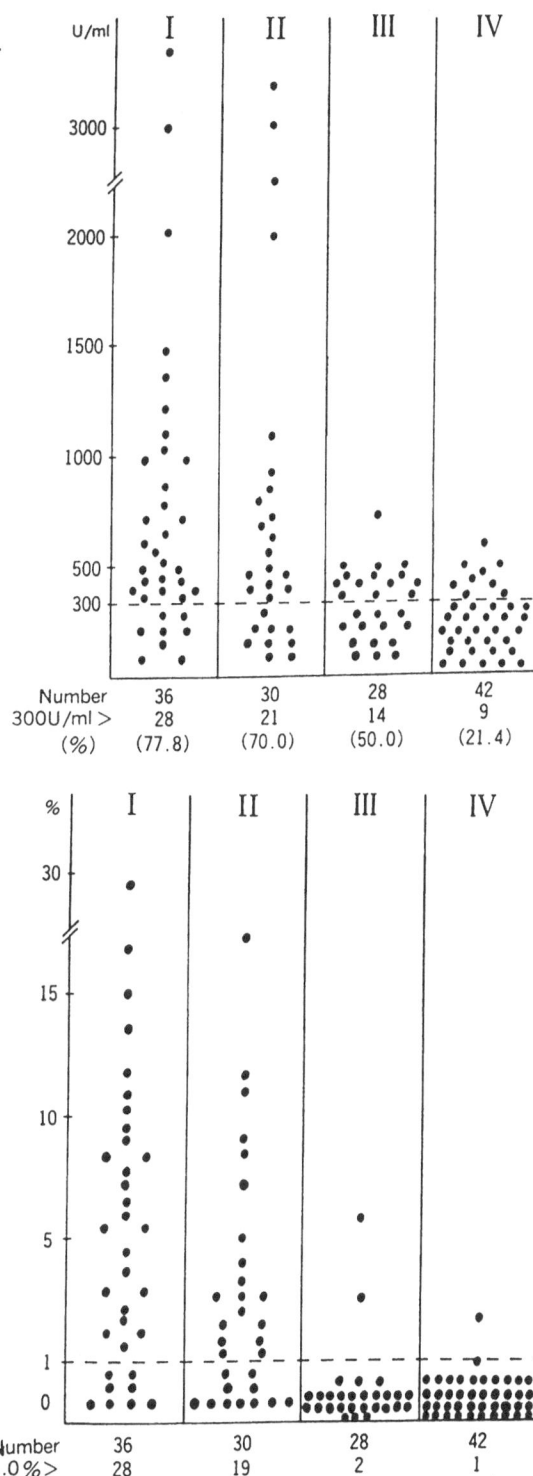

Fig. 2. Distribution of specific
IgE values in each group. A significant difference in specific IgE
rate was seen between types I and
II and types III and IV. Even
when detected, the values were
low in types III and IV

lishing an allergic condition in anisakiasis [11].

As a clinical sign of gastric anisakiasis, the focal site of pain is limited to the epigastrium. Therefore, it appears necessary in the diagnosis of severe epigastralgia accompanied by nausea, vomiting, together with considerations for acute gastritis, gastric ulcer, cholelithiasis, etc. that a differential diagnosis for gastric anisakiasis be included here in Japan.

Since anisakiasis is a benign disease, even in acute cases, symptomatic treatment of 2–10 days is sufficient to relieve the pain and this must be considered when surgery is planned.

References

1. Ishikura H (1978) Anisakiasis—Collecting edition and review of the literature in Japan. Hokkai Times, Sapporo, p 505 (in Japanese)
2. Ishikura H (1985) Anisakiasis, Review of the literature. (suppl) 1–6. p 139 (printed privately, in Japanese)
3. Ishikura H (1988) On anisakiasis: Survey of occurrence in the world and its pressing problems in Japan. Program of the 35th congress of Jpn. Gastroenterol. Endosc. May 26–28, 1988, Tokyo, p 123 (in Japanese)
4. Asaishi K, Nishino C, Totsuka M, Hayasaka H (1976) Eosinophilic inflammation of the alimentary canal caused by Anisakis larvae. Gastroenterol Surg 10: 405
5. Asaishi K, Nishino C, Totsuka M, Hayasaka H, Suzuki T (1980) Studies on the etiologic mechanism of anisakiasis: II. Epidemiologic study of inhabitants and questionaire survey in Japan. Jpn Soc Gastroenterol 15: 128
6. Nishino C (1977) Epidemiological studies on anisakiasis. Sapporo Med J 46: 73
7. Asaishi K (1974) Antigenic analysis of Anisakis larva and application of fluorescent antibody technique to histological diagnosis of anisakiasis. Sapporo Med J 43: 104
8. Sato Y, Yamashita T, Otsuru M, Suzuki T, Asaishi K, Nishino C (1975) Studies on the etiologic mechanism of anisakiasis: I. The anaphylactic reaction of digestive tract to the worm extracts. Jpn J Parasitol 24: 192
9. Asaishi K, Nishino C, Totsuka M, Hayasaka H, Suzuki T, Sato Y, Kenmotsu, Ohtsuru M (1978) Studies on the etiologic mechanism of anisakiasis: II. Antibody production of digestive tract induced by injection of the insolubled worm extracts. Jpn J Parasitol 27: 65
10. Asaishi K, Nishino C, Ebata T, Totsuka M, Hayasaka H, Suzuki T (1980) Studies on the etiologic mechanism of anisakiasis: I. Immunological reactions of digestive tract induced by Anisakis larva. Gastroenterol Jpn 15: 120
11. Saeki H (1975) Studies on cell-mediated immunity in experimental anisakiasis. Sapporo Med J 44: 309

Clinical Manifestation of Gastric Anisakiasis

H. Ohtaki and R. Ohtaki

Introduction

We diagnosed 72 patients in the Hokuriku district as having gastric anisakiasis following gastric fiberscope examination in our clinic over a 9-year period (January 1977 to December 1985). The patients were treated by removal of the larva in all cases. The clinical manifestations of gastric anisakiasis in these cases are described in this chapter. Van Thiel et al. [1] in 1960 first reported a patient suffering from acute abdominal pain caused by the *Anisakis* larva found in the intestine. Since then, many cases of anisakiasis have been reported. Most of the cases can be classified as the acute type on the basis of their clinical course with acute abdominal pain (acute type, fulminant form). However, in some cases, the pain is mild and lasts for a relatively long time (chronic type, mild form). There are also some cases in which patients without any severe symptoms are only later diagnosed as having gastric anisakiasis following endoscopic examination, as shown in the report of Hoshihara et al. [2]. In some cases, patients with acute abdominal pain did not undergo any endoscopic examination, and they were later diagnosed as having gastric anisakiasis as a result of endoscopic examination showing parasitic granuloma [3–6]. Even in the chronic type, close analysis of the patient's history reveals that most patients with gastric anisakiasis experienced some of the clinical symptoms, such as mild abdominal pain. These acute and chronic manifestations will be explained separately.

Case Report

Case 1: Severe Abdominal Pain

This was a 43-year-old male with severe abdominal pain brought in by ambulance. The patient had eaten raw mackerel at about 8 p.m. on the day prior to admission. He complained of epigastralgia that same night, with the pain becoming severe at 2 a.m. The pain did not decrease after the injection of a narcotic under the diagnosis of acute gastritis by the family doctor at 5 a.m. The patient experienced nausea and vomited twice.

The patient came to our hospital by ambulance at 7 a.m. as a result of the

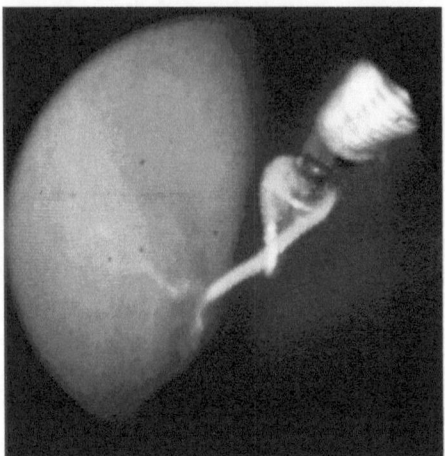

Fig. 1. Gastroendoscopic image showing removal the of *Anisakis* larva forceps

intolerable pain. There was no abnormality found upon urinalysis, and there was no anemia or leukocytoris upon admission. Diagnosis of gastric anisakiasis was made after history taking. Gastrofiberscopy was performed immediately and a larva of *Anisakis* was removed from the posterior wall of the gastric body (Fig. 1).

Case 2: Case of Hematemesis

The patient, a 50-year-old male, suffered epigastralgia at midnight and the pain gradually increased. The patient felt nausea and vomited twice, showing small amounts of hematemesis at 5 a.m. At 8 a.m. he consulted a doctor. His temperature was 36.8°C. No trouble was evident upon urinalysis or blood analysis. The result of examination was acute gastric mucosal lesion (AGML). We found gastric anabrosis, erosion, and bleeding, as shown in Fig. 2, by means of a gastric fiberscope. The patient, however, could not tolerate the instrument and it had to be removed temporarily. Thirty minutes, later we found a larva of *Anisakis* on the ruga gastrics of the greater curvature and removed it under the gastric fiberscope.

The patient had eaten marinated mackerel prior to the epigastralgia. In this case, the AGML occurred as the fulminant form of gastric anisakiasis.

Case 3: A type of mucosal tumor

The patient, a 36-year-old male, visited our clinic at midnight, as a result of severe epigastralgia. He experienced nausea, vomiting, and showed urticaria formation. There was no fever. The results of urinalysis were normal, and the red blood cell count was 48×10^4, white blood cell count 11 200, and hemoglobin 13.2 g/dl. A barium-filled X-ray film showed a tumor formation at the antrum. (Fig. 3). Fiberscopy was performed the following day (Fig. 4). Swelling of the mucus and stenosis of the antrum were revealed.

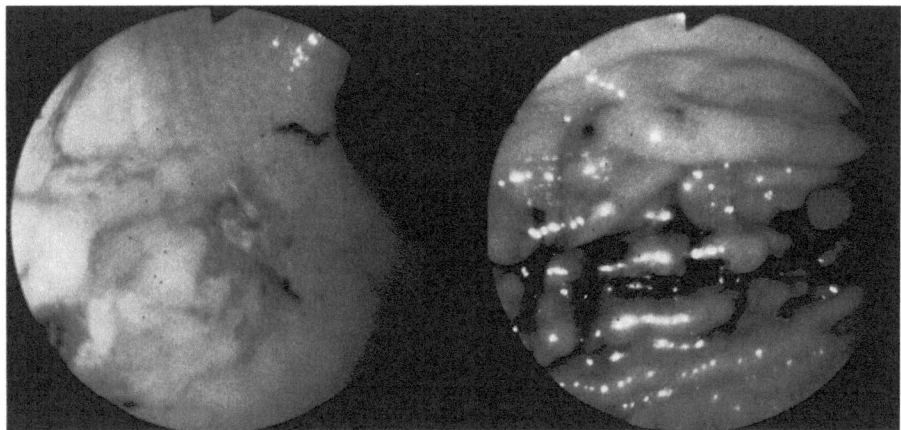

Fig. 2. Gastroendoscopic image showing a hemorrhagic lesion in case 2

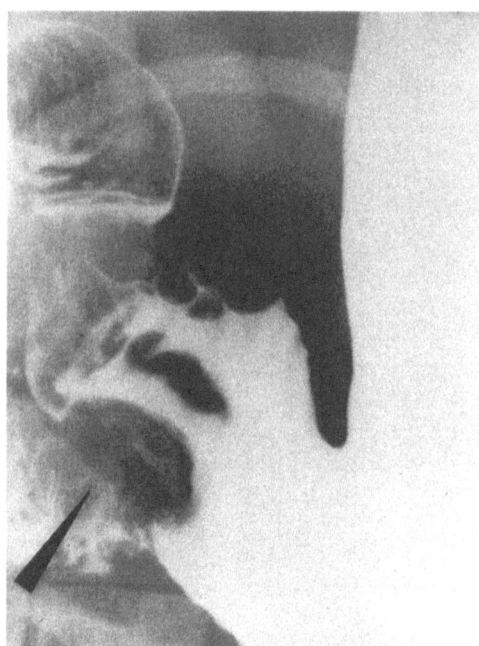

Fig. 3. Barium-filled X-ray image showing a filling defect in the antrum of the stomach in case 3

A gastric fiberscope could not be inserted to the prepyloric portion. So we, therefore, used a direct-vision endoscope along with the contrast-dye method. An *Anisakis* larva was then found beyond the mucous fold and removed (Fig. 5). Precise history taking showed that the patient had eaten marinated mackerel the previous day.

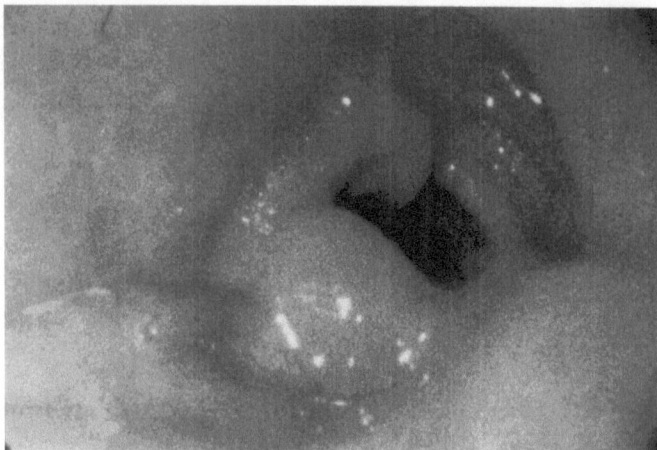

Fig. 4. Gastroendoscopic showing a protuberant lesion in the pyloric ring in case 3

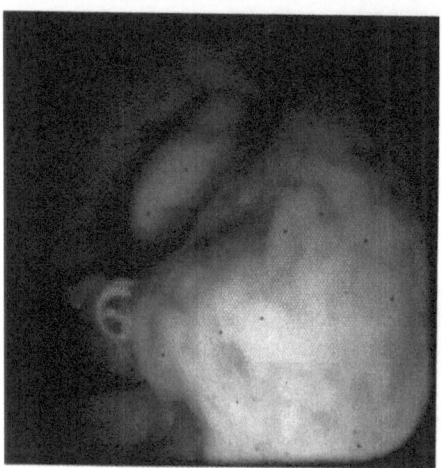

Fig. 5. Gastroendoscopic showing *Anisakis* larva beyond the proteuberant lesion in the pyloric ring in case 3

Clinical Manifestations of Gastric Anisakiasis

Acute (Fulminant) Type

Abdominal pain. Abdominal pain was experienced in all cases (Fig. 6), and occurred about 3–5 h after eating raw fish. Since Japanese often eat fish for supper, many patients complained of sudden acute abdominal pain late at night. The severity of the pain varied, ranging from mild to severe abdominal pain. In eight cases, patients were admitted late at night, complaining of severe ab-

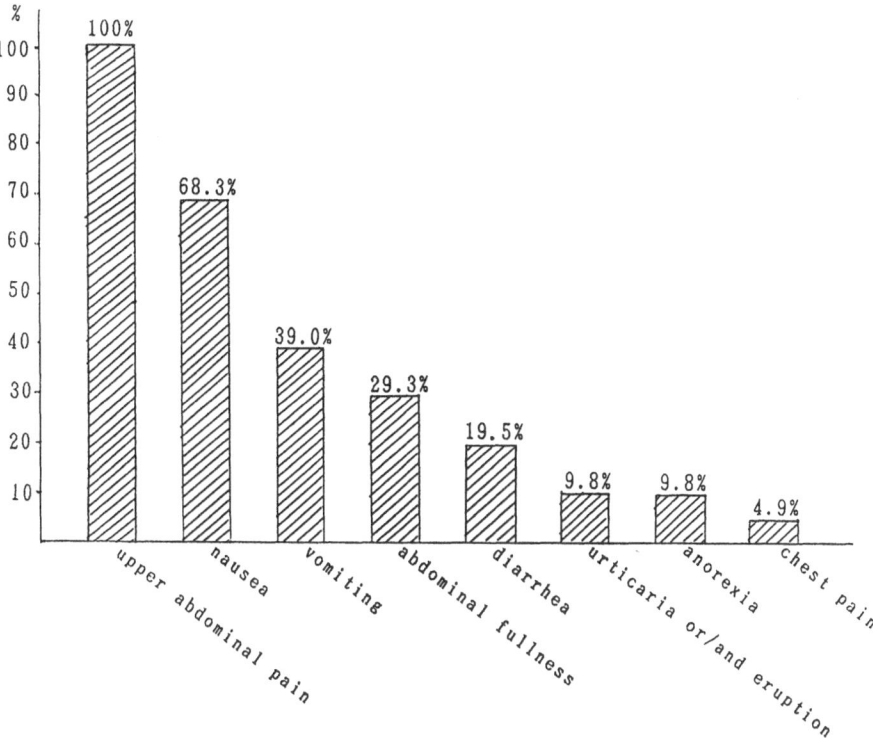

Fig. 6. Incidence of clinical symptoms of gastric anisakiasis (72 cases; January 1977 to December 1985)

dominal pain; two were admitted by ambulance (case 1). The other patients consulted their physicians during the daytime.

The time from onset until the first examination is listed in Table 1. Physicians were consulted within 24 h after the onset in 58 of 72 patients (about 80%). The region of pain was as follows: whole abdomen (40%), upper abdomen (50%), lower abdomen (10%). Patients with lower abdominal pain and diarrhea sometimes seem to have complications of intestinal anisakiasis.

As many researchers [7–15] suggest, abdominal pain is one of the most typical clinical manifestations and is sometimes treated surgically under the diagnosis of acute abdomen.

Nausea and vomiting. Nausea (68.3%) and vomiting (39%) were often observed with the abdominal pain. Most patients vomited the food contents only. However, in five cases, hematoemesis was also observed. In these cases, patients showed severe abdominal pain and consulted physicians within 6 h of the attack. Patients with severe hematoemesis were sometimes misdiagnosed as having a gastric ulcer and treated surgically by gastrectomy [16–18].

Table 1. Time from onset of symptoms until first examination

Time (h)	No. of cases
<6	8
<12	26
<24	24
<48	8
<96	6
Total	72

Abdominal distention. Abdominal distention was observed in about 30% of cases. The region mostly reported was the upper abdomen, but sometimes the whole abdomen was affected. Some of the abdominal distention could be defined under the umbilical region.

Diarrhea. Diarrhea was observed in 19.5% of the patients. Watery diarrhea occurred two to three times daily. One patient complained of episodes of diarrhea six times a day.

Urticaria. Some patients had urticaria or eruption (about 10%). The region reported involved was the chest, abdomen, and whole body. This is thought to be caused by an allergic mechanism caused by the larva.

Anorexia. Anorexia was observed in about 10% of the patients with abdominal pain and nausea. It is thought to be caused by accompanying gastritis.

Chest pain. Chest pain was observed in 49% of the patients reported as an uncomfortable dull pain.

The period of time from onset until the first examination is listed in Table 1. Besides the clinical symptoms mentioned above, some objective findings were also examined: (a) fever; (b) leukocytosis; (c) low erythrocyte sedimentation rate; (d) eosinophilia. These will be briefly described in the following.

Fever. In 7 of 62 cases, a slight fever was observed, with a temperature of about 37.5°C. High fever was noticed in only one case accompanied with colitis as reported by Ishikura.

Leukocytosis. In 40 of 53 cases, leukocytosis was observed: slight (9000–11 000/mm) 24.2%; moderate (11 000–13 000/mm) 12.1%; or severe (13 000–18 000/mm) 12.1%. There was no case showing leukocytosis above 18 000/mm.

Erythrocyte sedimentation rate. In none of 33 cases the erythrocyte sedimentation rate (ESR) was accelerated more than 10 mm/h.

Eosinophilia. Eosinophilia was found in 10 of 30 patients (8%–11% of eosinophils).

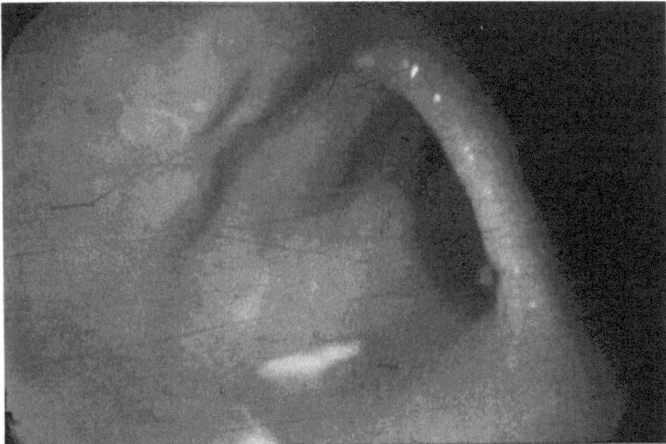

Fig. 7. Gastroendoscopic image showing *Anisakis* larva. The patient (35-year-old female) had severe abdominal pain 1 day after eating raw mackerel

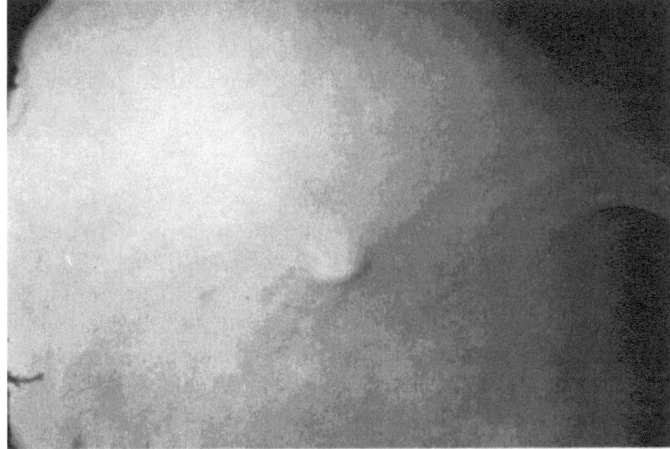

Fig. 8. Gastroendoscopic image after 1 month showing granulomatous change

Chronic (Mild) Type

In asymptomatic anisakiasis, it is difficult to make an accurate diagnosis. For example, a patient with abdominal pain who ate raw fish infected by an *Anisakis* larva 2 months previously will be difficult to diagnose. In one case, where there was no endoscope equipped with forceps, the diagnosis of gastric anisakiasis could be made by endoscopic examination but not treated. As shown in Fig. 7, an *Anisakis* larva was observed in the anterior wall of the gastric antrum. In this case, severe abdominal pain lasted for several days and dull abdominal pain was felt for about 2–3 months. Endoscopic observations after 1 month showed a

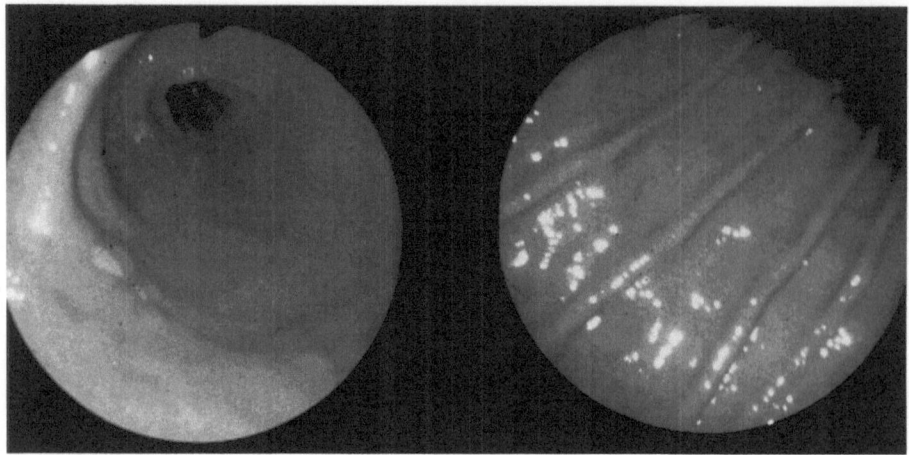

Fig. 9. Gastroendoscopic image showing an acute gastric ulcer

granuloma formation in the same lesion, as shown in Fig. 8. In this case, nausea and anorexia were also observed for a month in addition to dull abdominal pain.

Discussion

As clinicians, we frequently examine patients with acute gastric diseases. It is important to distinguish gastric anisakiasis from AGML, which may be caused by other factors. In this view, endoscopic examination would seem to be a requisite for accurate diagnosis. A patient with severe abdominal pain showing the AGML changes upon endoscopic examination, however, cannot be diagnosed as having gastric anisakiasis, unless an *Anisakis* larva is found. There was also a case in which one patient had the AGML changes and a history of eating raw fish but the larva became detached. In such a case, the diagnosis may be confusing.

As shown in Fig. 2 (case 2), a patient with severe epigastralgia was once diagnosed as having AGML from endoscopic examination. In this case, the *Anisakis* larva could not be found owing to the bleeding, but 1 h later endoscopic reexamination confirmed the existence of the larva and the final diagnosis of gastric anisakiasis was made. Nine days after the onset, the hemorrhagic lesion was treated, but it progressed into an acute gastric ulcer, as shown in Fig. 9.

Stress, drugs, raw fish, and alcohol consumption are all factors to be considered in AGML. The important point is that gastric anisakiasis is diagnosed only when the *Anisakis* larva can be identified. The diagnosis of anisakiasis is, therefore, not reliable if it is made only on the basis of history and symptoms but should be made by identification of the larva by endoscopic examination.

We studied 72 cases of gastric anisakiasis. We have also experienced the following: (a) Patients with upper abdominal pain and a history of eating raw fish who did not undergo endoscopic examination; (b) patients whose gastric X-ray film showed the typical signs of the presence of an *Anisakis* larva but who refused endoscopic examination; (c) patients who had upper abdominal pain and a history of eating raw fish but were not diagnosed as having gastric anisakiasis upon endoscopic examination, which showed the typical lesion of AGML. Figures 3–5 show a protuberant lesion in the gastric antrum. The condition was later diagnosed as gastric anisakiasis by endoscopic examination. The diagnosis of gastric anisakiasis is not always easy, so careful endoscopic examination by a specialist in endoscopy is required.

The incidence of gastric ulcer or gastric cancer with gastric anisakiasis is rare although there are some reports [20, 21]. As pointed out by Ishikura [22], gastric anisakiasis can sometimes be misdiagnosed as gastric ulcer, gastric cancer, gastric polyp, duodenal ulcer, or cholelithiasis. However, recent progress in the techniques of endoscopic examination and a positive attitude toward endoscopic examination even in the acute phase of gastric mucosal lesion have markedly decreased the incidence of misdiagnosis.

Summary

We have experienced 72 cases of gastric anisakiasis. Most patients had a history of eating raw fish with clinical manifestations, such as acute abdominal pain. They were diagnosed and treated by endoscopic examination. However, in some cases such as the hemorrhagic type (case 2) or the tumorous type (case 3), final diagnosis was very difficult. The possibility of gastric anisakiasis must be taken into consideration with patients suffering from acute abdominal pain, particularly when there is a history of regular consumption of raw fish. Prompt endoscopic examination is necessary for accurate diagnosis and treatment.

References

1. Van Thiel PH, Kuipers FC, Roskam RT (1960) A nematode parasitic to herring causing acute abdominal syndromes in man. Trop Geogr Med 12: 97–113
2. Hoshihara Y, Yamamoto T, Koyama M, Kawahara H, Kawaguchi Y, Watanabe K (1984) A case of gastric anisakiasis without acute gastrointestinal symptoms, unexpectedly found by contrast dye-method on the endoscopic examination. Progr Digest Endoscop 25: 223–225 (in Japanese)
3. Kihara T, Tsuji O, Tanikawa T, Asakura A, Sakumoto D (1968) A case of submucosal gastric tumor. Stomach Intestine 3: 457–461 (in Japanese)
4. Iino H, Tomioka T, Akaiwa J, Mochizuki S, Soh N (1969) Parasitic granuloma of the stomach—Gastric anisakiasis and larva of Anisakis. Stomach Intestine 4: 601–608 (in Japanese)
5. Ishiyama I, Yoshitake Y, Sumida S (1970) A case of gastric anisakiasis associated with erosive gastritis. Stomach Intestine 5: 373–377 (in Japanese)
6. Ohmori H, Kimoto K, Nanba T, Hanabusa H, Sugimoto S, Watanabe H, Ohtaki H, Matsuura H, Tanabe T, Kibayashi H, Kurihara M, Okajima K (1979) A case of gastric anisakiasis showing interesting findings. Stomach Intestine 14: 977–981 (in Japanese)
7. Namiki M, Morooka T, Kawauchi H, Ueda N, Sekiya C, Nakagawa K, Furuta T, Ohguro T, Kamata H (1970) The diagnosis of acute gastric anisakiasis. Stomach

Intestine 5: 1437–1440 (in Japanese)

8. Kawauchi H, Namiki T, Morooka T, Nakagawa K, Ohguro T (1973) Gastric anisa-kiasis presenting acute gastrointestinal symptoms. Stomach Intestine 8: 31–38 (in Japanese)
9. Ishikura H (1969) Occurrence of anisakiasis and its clinical presentation. Saishin Igaku 24: 357–365 (in Japanese)
10. Ohtaki H, Ohtaki R, Ohtaki T, Nakaya H (1982) Clinical study of anisakiasis diagnosed and treated by endoscopy. Scand J Gastroenterol 17: [Suppl 78] 66
11. Ohtaki H, Nitta T, Tanikawa K, Tsukioka T, Shimazaki S (1980) Clinical study of AGML and gastric anisakiasis. Jpn J Prim Care 2: 313–317 (in Japanese)
12. Hanamure B (1980) Studies on 27 cases of gastric anisakiasis by endoscopic examina-tion. Gastroenterol Endosc 22: 592 (in Japanese)
13. Yoshimura H, Kondo K, Ohnishi Y, Akao N, Tsubota N (1978) Summary of the patients with anisakiasis for the past three years, with special reference to clinico-pathology and immuno-diagnosis. Jpn Med J 2837: 29–32 (in Japanese)
14. Fukumoto S, Yoshida H, Ashizawa N, Shizuku N, Yamashita H, Ryu S, Nishimura K, Ikeda T, Watanabe M, Hirakawa H, Shimada N (1983) Clinical study of acute anisakiasis. Jpn Gastroenterol 80: 695 (in Japaese)
15. Asaishi K, Nishino C, Totsuka M, Hayasaka H, Suzuki T (1980) Studies on the etiologic mechanism of anisakiasis: II. Epidemiologic study of inhabitants and ques-tionaire survey in Japan. J Jpn Soc Gastroenterol 15: 128–134
16. Ito S, Kishi S, Kimura M, Seki H, Kitamura Y, Urakami Y, Ishikawa K, Akagi G, Izuki T (1973) Report of two cases of gastric anisakiasis—Removal of living anisakis larva out of ulcer floor. Stomach Intestine 8: 1375–1380 (in Japanese)
17. Mori R, Hirai Y, Fukushima H, Nagamatsu S, Ohe H, Murakami M, Ohta Y, Eguchi M, Tokuyasu K (1980) A case of gastric anisakiasis with mass hematoemesis. J Jpn Soc Int Med 69: 381 (in Japanese)
18. Shinno T, Watanabe K, Yoshimura H, Akao N (1982) A case of gastric anisakiasis with hematoemesis. Jpn J Gastroenterol 79: 1544 (in Japanese)
19. Yokoya H, Ohe K, Miyoshi A, Hidaka T, Murakami Y, Tsuji M (1980) Three cases of acute gastric anisakiasis—especially of its seroimmunological diagnosis. Stomach Intestine 15: 1329–1335 (in Japanese)
20. Iino H (1985) Anisakiasis in Kyushu. Gastroenterol Endoscopy 27: 630 (in Japanese)
21. Hoshihara Y, Tsubura K, Yamamoto T, Watanabe K, Koyama M, Kawaguchi Y, Kawahara H (1986) Three cases of gastric anisakiasis. Gastroenterol Endoscopy 28: 451 (in Japanese)
22. Ishikura H (1978) Anisakiasis. Hokkai Times, Sapporo (in Japanese)

Endoscopic Findings of Gastric Anisakiasis with Acute Symptoms

M. Namiki and Y. Yazaki

Namiki et al. [1, 2] and Kawauchi et al. [3] performed urgent endoscopic examinations on patients showing acute gastric symptoms such as epigastric pain and nausea 4–6 h after the patients had eaten fresh marine products. *Anisakis* larvae were observed penetrating the gastric wall; the worms were removed endoscopically with biopsy forceps and identified parasitologically as *Anisakis simplex* larva. Since these advances in 1968, the disease has become the cause of wide concern in Japan. Cases with *Pseudoterranova decipiens* larva were later found to show similar symptoms to those of cases with *Anisakis* larvae type I [4, 5]. In both cases, the mechanism involved is thought to be an allergic reaction induced in the submucosal layer of the gastric wall around the penetration site of the worm [6]. Endoscopic findings of gastric anisakiasis are described in the present chapter.

Endoscopic Findings at Penetration Site and Adjacent Area

Care should be taken not to mistake the worm penetrating the gastric wall for the stringlike mucus. As seen on closer observation, an *Anisakis* larva shows a thin, stringlike appearance and its color is milk-white, while a *Pseudoterranova decipiens* larva is broader and yellow or yellowish-brown in color [5]. In the early phase of penetration into the gastric wall, the worm moves actively, showing fast winding movements. In addition, the worm shows various forms, i.e., a coiled form and a sigmoid form (Figs. 1, 2). Later, the worm moves slowly and becomes loosely stretched (Fig. 3). Most penetration sites are edematous to varying degrees, sometimes accompanied with redness. Erosion and bleeding are observed in some cases. It is not difficult to locate the worm by looking for such an edematous and/or reddish gastric mucosa in cases suspected of the disease. A case was reported of a submucosal tumor with a central depressive area measuring 15 × 15 mm observed 3 weeks after the onset of symptoms. Subsequently, an eosinophilic granuloma was revealed with a dead *Anisakis* larva at its center in the resected stomach [7]. Therefore, removal of the worm from the gastric wall is necessary.

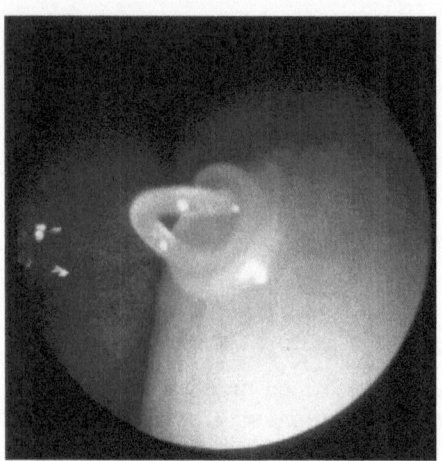

Fig. 1. An *Anisakis simplex* larva, showing the coiled form

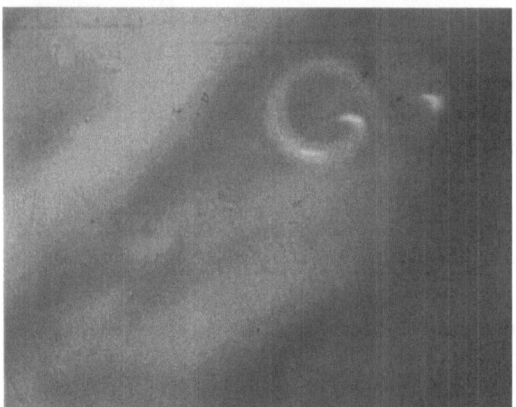

Fig. 2. An *Anisakis simplex* larva, showing the sigmoid form

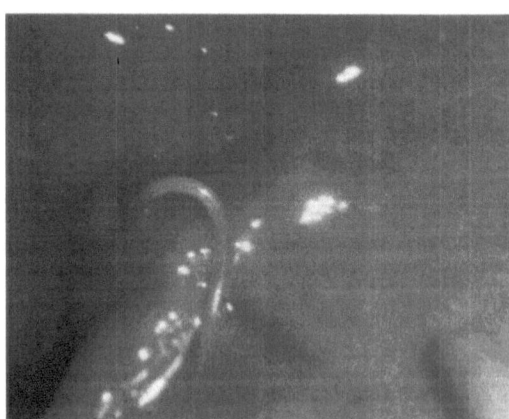

Fig. 3. An *Anisakis simplex* larva observed 13 days after the onset of symptoms. Note the loosely stretched form of the worm

Fig. 4. An *Anisakis simplex* larva penetrating the edematous longitudinal gastric mucosal fold

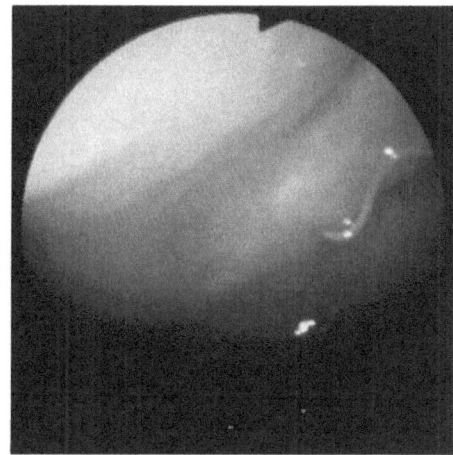

Endoscopic Findings in Other Parts of Gastric Mucosa

The gastric mucosa other than the penetration site often shows broad edematous changes and some cases may be misdiagnosed as Borrmann type 4 gastric cancer. Thickening of the longitudinal gastric mucosal folds with edematous changes caused by the penetration of the worm could be seen in some cases (Fig. 4). Sometimes, the worm moving in the stomach without penetrating the stomach wall is observed (Fig. 5). Many erosions and red spots are observed, mainly in the antrum of the stomach, in some cases; these lesions may be caused by further penetrations of the worm wandering about in the stomach [5] and/or other secondary changes.

Penetration Sites of the Worm

The *Anisakis* larva is reported to penetrate not only the gastric wall but also the mucous membrane of the larynx [8], esophagus, duodenum, small intestine terminal portion of the ileum), and colon.

In other words, it is likely that the worm can penetrate any part of the digestive tract. The incidence of penetration of the worm, however, is low except in the stomach. Of the 238 cases of penetration of the worm in the upper digestive tract we have experienced, there was one case in the bulbus of the duodenum and another in the lower part of esophagus; all the other were in the stomach. The most frequent penetration site in the stomach was around the greater curvature of the posterior wall of the middle corpus. More than one worm was sometimes found to have penetrated the stomach. Therefore, care should be taken not to overlook additional worms. We experienced one case in which four *Anisakis simplex* larvae had penetrated the gastric wall.

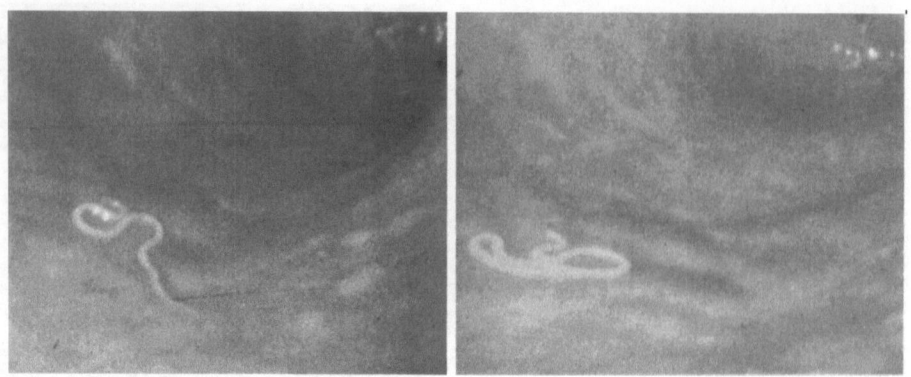

a   b

Fig. 5a, b. An *Anisakis simplex* larva detached from the gastric wall, wandering around in the stomach

Associated Gastric Diseases

Of the 238 cases of gastric anisakiasis we have experienced, we observed two cases accompanied with gastric cancer (type IIc early gastric cancer and Borrmann type 2 gastric cancer), four with a gastric ulcer, and two with a duodenal ulcer. The relationship between these diseases and gastric anisakiasis is unknown. It is of interest that the worms were found to be penetrating the ulcerative area in two cases with gastric ulcer and two with gastric cancer.

The endoscopic findings of gastric anisakiasis with acute symptoms can thus be summarized as follows:
a) Penetration site
   1) Edema
   2) Redness
   3) Erosion
   4) Bleeding
b) Other part of the stomach
   1) Generalized edema
   2) Edema of longitudinal gastric mucosal folds
   3) Erosive gastritis
   4) Presence of the worm only (not penetrated)
   5) No changes
c) Associated gastric diseases
   1) Gastric cancer (IIc, Borrmann 2)
   2) Gastric ulcer

References

1. Namiki M, Morooka T, Kawauchi H, Ueda N, Sekiya C, Nakagawa K (1969) Endoscopic observation of anisakis larvae in the stomach and some interesting findings. Gastroenterol Endoscopy 12: 302 (in Japanese)

2. Namiki M, Morooka T, Kawauchi H, Kawauchi H, Ueda N, Sekiya C, Nakagawa K, Furuta T, Oguro T, Kamada H (1970) Diagnosis of acute gastric anisakiasis. Stomach Intestine 5: 1437–1440 (in Japanese)
3. Kawauchi H, Namiki M, Morooka T, Nakagawa K, Oguro T (1973) Gastric anisakiasis presenting acute gastrointestinal symptoms—With special references to the endoscopic and roentgenographic findings of anisakis larva penetrating into the wall of the human stomach and to its clinical features. Stomach Intestine 8: 31–38 (in Japanese)
4. Nagano K, Takagi K, Yanagawa I, Ohishi K, Kagei N (1973) Acute heterocheilidasis of the stomach (due to terranova decipiens). Stomach Intestine 8: 81–85 (in Japanese)
5. Doi K, (1973) Clinical aspects of acute heterocheilidasis of the stomach (due to larvae of anisakis and terranova decipiens)—Especially on its differential diagnosis by X-ray and endoscopy. Stomach Intestine 8: 1513–1518 (in Japanese)
6. Suzuki T, Ishikura H (1974) Pathogenic mechanisms, symptoms and diagnosis of anisakiasis. Fishes and Anisakis (No. 7 fisheries scientific series). The Japanese Society of Scientific Fisheries. Kohseisha kohseikaku, Tokyo, pp 58–72 (in Japanese)
7. Okada K, Tsuchiya M, Tanaka N, Hashizume Y (1978) A case of acute anisakiasis of the stomach making rapid progress to parasitic granuloma. Progr Digest Endoscopy 12: 153–155 (in Japanese)
8. Nishimura T, Tanaka E, Ito Y, Sugihara Y, Morishita K, Watanabe S, Watanabe Sachiko (1974) Report of three cases of human anisakiasis: Larvae, each recovered from the different organs of men, and their morphological studies. J Hyogo Med College 2: 124–137 (in Japanese)

Acute Gastric Anisakiasis with Special Analysis of the Location of the Worms Penetrating the Gastric Mucosa

O. Shibata, Y. Uchida, and T. Furusawa

Introduction

A clinical feature of acute gastric anisakiasis is that diagnostic and therapeutic procedures can be performed simultaneously by endoscopically extracting the parasites by using forceps. It is important, therefore, to investigate the predisposing site of penetration of *Anisakis* larvae through the gastric mucous membrane.

Materials and Methods

A total of 258 cases with acute gastric anisakiasis were treated at Furusawa Gastrointestinal Hospital for a period of 9 years from 1977 to 1985. In these cases, a total of 274 parasites could be endoscopically extracted with forceps; except for five, they were identified parasitologically as *Anisakis simplex* larva. Both radiological and endoscopic examinations were carried out simultaneously in 190 of the 258 cases. As for the remaining 68 cases, only endoscopic examinations were performed. The sites at which the parasites were endoscopically extracted were plotted on a map of the stomach developed with the greater curvature incised. The stomach was divided into four parts—anterior wall, lesser curvature, posterior wall, and greater curvature. It was further divided along the long axis into the cardiac region, fornix, upper body, middle body, lower body, angulus, antrum, and pyloric regions. An analytical study was made of the relation between the sites of parasitic penetration and the radiological and endoscopic findings.

Results

Sites of Parasite-Penetration

The sites of penetration of the endoscopically extracted parasites are shown in Fig. 1. There were 14 cases in which two parasites were extracted and one case in which three were extracted. Thus, a total of 274 parasites were extracted from

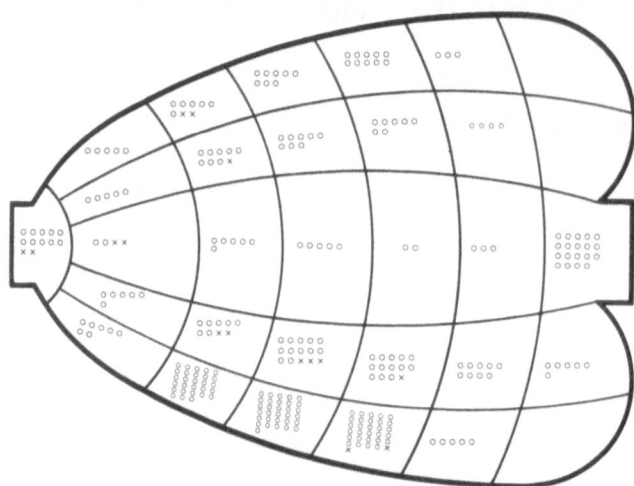

Fig. 1. Location of the *Anisaki simplex* larvae penetrating the gastric mucosa (258 cases; 1977–1985). *Circles* represent worms, *crosses* additional worms in the same stomach

the 258 cases. When two or more parasites were observed in the same patient, the one penetrating the oral side was indicated by a white dot, and the other by a cross. In terms of the map distribution with the stomach divided into four parts, as many as 129 parasites (48%) were found in the greater curvature. This was followed by 61 (22%) in the posterior wall, 33 (11%) in the anterior wall, and 20 (7%) in the lesser curvature (Table 1). With respect to the distribution with the stomach divided along the long axis, the largest number of parasites, 45, was found in the middle body greater curvature. This was followed by 34 in the lower body greater curvature and 31 in the angulus greater curvature. In the middle body lesser curvature, there were only two parasites.

Gastric X-ray Findings

Gastric X-ray examinations were conducted in 190 cases, and the following findings were obtained for acute gastric anisakiasis: (a) Edematous hypertrophic folds, 184 cases (96%); (b) failure to depict the antrum area due to compressed picture, 156 cases (82%); (c) visualization of parasites, 120 cases (63%); (d) opening of gastric angulus, 115 cases (60%). The relation between the site of parasitic penetration and the opening of the gastric angulus is shown in Table 2. The opening of the gastric angulus was observed at a rate of 100% in cases with parasitic penetration in the lesser curvature of the antrum, lower, middle, and upper bodies, and in the anterior wall of the middle body. It was observed at a rate of 70% or more in cases with parasitic penetration in the lower body anterior wall, upper body greater curvature, cardiac region, and lower body posterior wall. It was noteworthy that the opening of the gastric angulus was observed in 94% of the cases with penetration in the lesser curvature as against 48% of those in the greater curvature. A specific gastroroentgenographic feature was that the opening of the gastric angulus was noted in 11 of 14 cases (79%) with penetration in the cardiac region.

Table 1. Worms (total 274) penetrating the gastric mucosa (258 cases); 1977–1985

Location	Anterior wall	Lesser curvature	Posterior wall	Greater curvature	Other	Total
Pyrolic region	—	—	—	—	12	12
Antrum	5	4	7	11	—	27
Angulus	10	6	9	31	—	56
Lower body	8	5	15	34	—	62
Middle body	6	2	14	45	—	67
Upper body	4	3	9	8	—	24
Fornix	—	—	7	—	—	7
Cardiac region	—	—	—	—	19	19
Total	33	20	61	129	31	274

Endoscopic Findings

The endoscopic features of acute gastric anisakiasis were as follows: (a) Existence of *Anisakis* larvae; (b) edematous hypertrophic gastric folds; (c) increase of gastric secretion and gastric peristalsis; (d) the findings of mucosal lesions through which *Anisakis* larvae penetrated were as follows: 120 cases (46%) of edema, 64 cases (25%) of redness, 48 cases (19%) of coagulation, 16 cases (6%) of hemorrhage, and ten (4%) cases of ulceration; (e) erosions in the other gastric mucosa were seen at a smaller incidence than erosive gastrtis.

Edematous hypertrophic gastric folds were observed along the long axis of the stomach, primarily occurring on the side of greater curvature. The folds numbered one in 69 cases (27%), two in 116 cases (45%), and three in 52 cases (20%). Thus, in the largest number of cases there were two folds. With regard to the site of parasitic penetration in connection with edematous hypertrophic gastric folds, there were as many as 196 cases (76%) with penetration on the oral side, 32 cases (12%) in the middle portion, 25 cases (10%) on the anal side, and five cases (2%) having local swelling.

Discussion

A total of 258 cases with acute gastric anisakiasis were treated, and 274 parasites were extracted over a 9-year period at Furusawa Gastrointestinal Hospital. This chapter is primarily concerned with the relation between the predisposing site of parasitic penetration and radiological and endoscopic findings.

Reports on the site of parasitic penetration available in Japan are listed in Table 3. When the stomach is divided into three parts as in this table, the incidence of penetration was highest in the body, followed by, respectively, the antrum, cardia, and fornix.

In the case of dividing the stomach into four parts—anterior wall, lesser curvature, posterior wall, and greater curvature—the incidence of penetration was found to be highest in the greater curvature, where it was much higher than in the lesser curvature (Table 4).

Table 2. Relation between the location and the opening of the angle in the radiological findings (190 cases)

Location	No. of cases	Anterior wall	Lesser curvature	Posterior wall	Greater curvature	Other	Total
Pyloric region	5	—	—	—	—	3/5	3/5 (60)
Antrum	22	2/5 (40)	2/2(100)	3/6 (50)	4/9 (44)	—	11/22 (50)
Angulus	38	5/7 (71)	3/4 (75)	3/5 (60)	10/22(50)	—	21/38 (55)
Lower body	47	7/8 (89)	5/5(100)	8/11(73)	12/23(52)	—	32/47 (68)
Middle body	40	5/5(100)	2/2(100)	5/8 (63)	25/10(40)	—	22/40 (55)
Upper body	19	3/4 (75)	3/3(100)	4/7 (57)	4/5 (80)	—	14/19 (74)
Fornix	5	—	—	—	—	1/5	1/5 (20)
Cardiac region	14	—	—	—	—	11/14	11/14 (79)
Total	190	22/29(76)	15/16(94)	23/37(62)	40/84(48)	—	115/190(60)

Figures in parentheses percentages

Table 3. Location of the worms reported in the literature with the stomach divided into three parts

Study	No. of worms	Antrum (%)	Body (%)	Cardia & fornix (%)
Kawauchi et al. [3]	48	17	80	—
Odawara et al. [4]	29	36	60	4
Kusuhara [5]	203	16	75	9
Fujino et al. [6]	157	22	68	11
Nagano [7]	140	14	58	28
Shibata et al.	274	14	76	9

Table 4. Location of the worms reported in the literature with the stomach divided into four parts

Study	No. of worms	Anterior wall (%)	Lesser curvature (%)	Posterior wall (%)	Greater curvature (%)
Kusuhara [5]	203	17	8	19	48
Fujino et al. [6]	155	24	6	32	37
Omachi et al. [8]	51	14	6	25	55
Nagano [7]	140	20	15	26	39
Shibata et al.	274	12	7	22	47

No paper has been published to our knowledge dealing with why *Anisakis* larvae are predominant on the side of the greater curvature of the body. It is reported that *Anisakis* larvae are strongly resistant to acid [1], and in this conjunction, it is suggested that there is a relation between the site of penetration and acid secretion by the gastric wall.

It should be noted that there are a larger number of folds and more active secretion of mucus on the side of the greater curvature. A valley between folds with a supply of mucus may afford a good environment for *Anisakis* larvae.

Opening of the gastric angulus was an important finding gastroroentgenologically, because it suggests parasitic penetration near the angulus, in particular on the side of lesser curvature [2]. Edematous hypertrophic gastric folds, found endoscopically, were noted along the longer axis of the stomach. There were some cases in which two or more folds were observed.

The parasites tended to penetrate mostly from the oral side of the folds. The local findings on penetration were obtained as edema at a rate of 46%. This obversation is worthy of attention.

A gastric X-ray film even erroneously suggested scirrhous carcinoma. Thus, the utmost care should be taken in making any diagnostic judgement.

Summary

The predisposing sites of parasitic penetration were the gastric middle body, lower body, and angulus on the side of greater curvature.

The parasites tend to penetrate from the oral side of edematous hypertrophic gastric folds. It is expedient, therefore, to look for them initially on the oral side of the folds.

References

1. Iino H, Tomioka T, Akaiwa J, Mochizuki A, Sou N (1969) Parasitic granuloma of the stomach-gastric anisakiasis and larva of anisakis. Stomach Intestine 4: 601–608 (in Japanese)
2. Shibata O, Ichimanda M, Furusawa T, Arita T, Kudo T, Emoto O (1981) Acute gastric anisakiasis—with special analysis of the roentgenographic findings. J Nagasaki Med Soc 56: 20–25 (in Japanese)
3. Kawauchi H, Namiki T, Morooka T, Nakagawa K, Oguro T (1973) Gastric anisakiasis presenting acute gastrointestinal symptoms—with special references to the endoscopic and roentgenographic findings of *Anisakis* larva penetrating into the wall of the human stomach and its clinical features. Stomach Intestine 8: 31–38 (in Japanese)
4. Odawara R, Nishi M, Nomura H, Aiko T, Kaneko Y, Kawaji T, Hagihara K, Kawaida S, Kodama T, Kasamo H, Maenohara S, Matsushita F, Makizumi S, Yoshimori M (1979) Acute anisakiasis of the stomach—in special reference to roentgenological diagnosis. Jpn J Gastrointestinal Surg 12: 257–263 (in Japanese)
5. Kusuhara T (1983) Clinical study of acute gastric anisakiasis: II. Radiological and endoscopical features. J Kumamoto Med Soc 57: 69–79 (in Japanese)
6. Fujino T, Ooiwa T, Ishii Y (1984) Clinical, epidemiological and morphological studies on 150 cases of acute gastric anisakiasis in Fukuoka prefecture. Jpn J Parasitol 33: 73–92 (in Japanese)
7. Nagano K (1985) The individual review of the heterocheilidiasis (as a synonym for the anisakiasis). J Donan Med Soc 20: 302–312 (in Japanese)
8. Omachi K, Omachi T, Maruyama Y (1985) Anisakiasis of gastrointestinal tract in Nagano prefecture. Shinsyu Med J 33: 42–56 (in Japanese)

Aspects of Mucosal Changes in Gastric Anisakiasis

T. OOIWA, K. SUGIMACHI, and M. MORI

Introduction

Acute gastric anisakiasis caused by mucosal penetration of *Anisakis* larvae is fairly common in Japan as many species of fish, including mackerel, are often eaten raw [1–3]. Hence in patients with acute epigastric pain, anisakiasis should always be considered.

As the larvae of *Anisakis* present in the gastric mucosa can be observed endoscopically, extraction is for the most part feasible [2]. The clinical features and characteristic findings at endoscopy and in upper gastrointestinal tract series plus the mucosal changes in gastric anisakiasis are described in this chapter.

Materials and Methods

Between December 1969 and March 1986, 213 patients with acute epigastric pain were diagnosed endoscopically as having acute gastric anisakiasis. Of these 213, 170 underwent an upper gastrointestinal (GI) tract series, using the conventional barium contrast method with patients in the recumbent and prone positions, with or without compression. The double-contrast method was commonly used. Valethamate bromide (10 mg), a spasmolytic, was routinely given to all of these patients to decrease gastric tonus.

All of the 213 patients underwent endoscopy and during this procedure representative photographs were taken prior to biopsy. The following types of endoscope were used: Olympus (1969–1978) GTF-B2; Olympus (1969–1978) GIF-D2; Olympus (1978–1985) GTF-B100; Olympus (1978–1985) GIF-Q; Olympus (after 1985) GF-10; and Olympus (after 1985) GIF-Q10.

All endoscopes were either forward or lateral viewing and uniformly equipped with a biopsy channel.

Once the larvae were identified, they were grasped with biopsy forceps and slowly pulled away from the mucosa through the biopsy channel. To avoid tearing, the flap of the biopsy channel was removed.

Upon removal, the *Anisakis* larvae were immediately fixed in 10% formalin and treated with petrolatum alcohol and lactophenol to increase the transparency for microscopic studies.

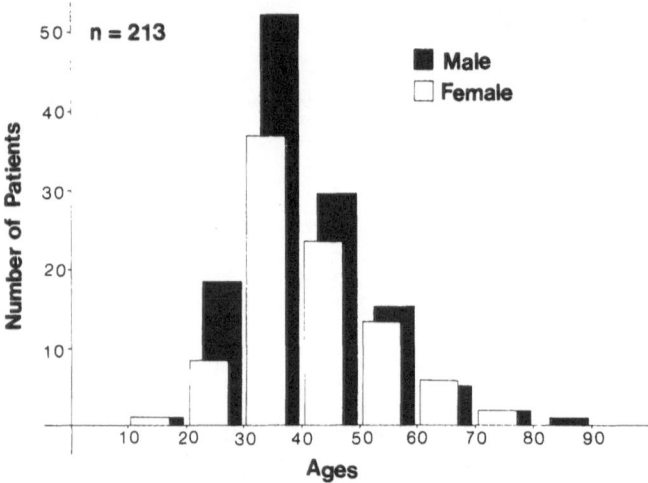

Fig. 1. Age distribution of 213 patients with acute gastric anisakiasis

All of the removed larvae were either stage III or stage IV *Anisakis simplex* larvae [3].

Results

All the patients were Japanese and included 122 men (57.2%) and 91 women (42.7%), ranging in age from 18 to 82 years (Fig. 1).

Mackerel was the fish most commonly eaten; the next most common were horse mackerel and sardines.

After eating the raw fish, the onset of symptoms was quite rapid. The larva was removed the same day in 52 patients, on the 2nd day in 79, and on the 3rd day in 64. In 89.2% of the patients, the larvae were removed by the 3rd day and all were removed by the 6th day at the very latest.

Subjective Symptoms

The most common symptom was severe epigastric pain, which occurred in all patients. The interval between eating the contaminated fish and development of symptoms ranged from 1 to 36 h, with 70% of the patients having the symptoms within 8 h.

The pain was usually described as colicky, located primarily in the epigastrium.

In 23 of the 213 patients, the symptoms were severe and parenteral analgesics and ambulance transportation to the hospital were required.

Severe epigastric pain was present in all 213 patients, nausea in 115 (54%), anorexia in 79 (35.7%), and emesis in 58 (27.2%).

Table 1. Roentgenographic findings in 140 patients

	No. of cases	Percent
Rigidity of margin		
Absent	37	26.4
Present		
Slight	84	60.0
Extensive	19	13.5
Edema of mucosa		
Absent	26	18.6
Present		
Partial	72	51.4
Widespread	42	30.0

Radiological Findings

Radiographic studies were performed in 140 patients prior to removal of the larvae. Threadlike gastric filling defects, approximately 30 mm in length, are characteristic of the disease. However, in 48 of these patients (34.3%), the larvae were clearly demonstrated on the X-ray. In another 16 patients, the larvae were faintly evident. The shape was usually circular or ringlike, and the shapes occasionally changed. The larvae of *Anisakis* become fixed at certain points, penetrate the mucosa, and may appear as a small, round collection of barium.

The larvae were more often identified when the gastric mucosa was well defined. Identification was often difficult when the mucosa was distorted by edema or obscured by mucus.

The distensibility of the stomach along the greater and lesser curvature was then examined. In 37 patients (26.4%), no abnormal finding was observed. An unnatural rigidity of the margin, dilatation of the angle, or narrowing of the antrum were observed in 84 patients (60%). Strong rigidity of the margin, accompanied by a filling defect or with markedly poor distensibility, was also seen in 19 patients (13.6%; Table 1).

Mucosal edema is usually present, hence the diagnosis may become difficult. An adequate compression technique, as well as a double-contrast study, aids in the identification of the larvae. In some cases, however, radiological demonstration is hampered because of this edema. A swelling of the gastric folds, particularly in the double-contrast image, was also considered characteristic of the edema. If no abnormality was present on the compression and double-contrast films, then edema was assumed to be zero. Partial edema was defined as the presence of an ill-defined defect present on the compression film or when localized swollen and prominent folds were seen on the double-contrast film. Widespread edema was defined as a more diffuse pattern which involved almost the entire gastric corpus. The resulting marked deformity could possibly be mistaken for rigidity.

Using these criteria, no edema was seen in 12 patients (8.6%), partial edema of the mucosa noted in 86 (61.4%), and widespread edema observed in 42 (30%).

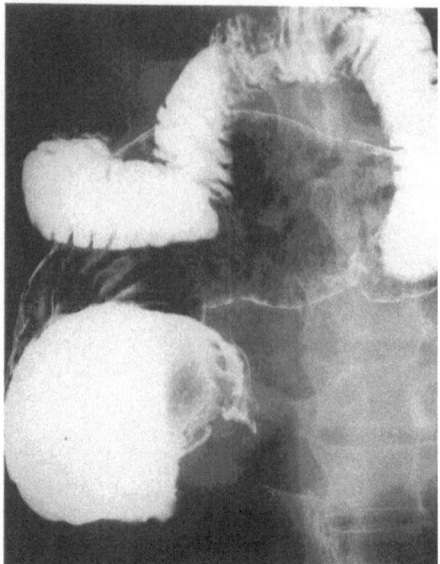

Fig. 2. Roentgenographic findings. Note the "vanishing tumor" of the gastric cardia. This tumor rapidly disappeared after endoscopic removal of the larvae

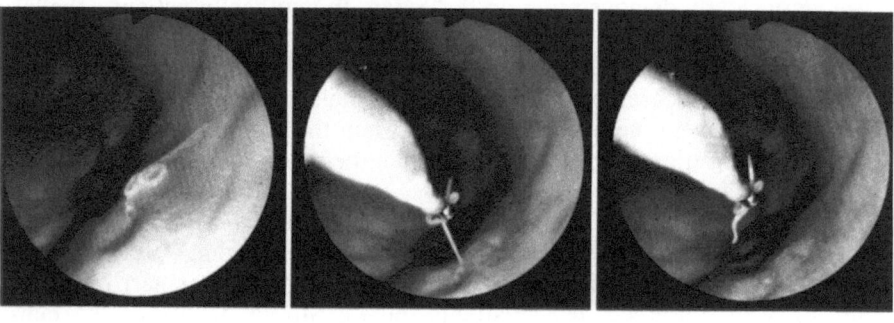

a   b, c

Fig. 3a–c. Endoscopic findings. **a** An *Anisakis* larva is found in the flat mucosa of the stomach; **b** it is then grasped and **c** removed with biopsy forceps

In a few cases, the lesion revealed the so-called vanishing tumor [4], which rapidly disappeared after endoscopic removal of the larvae (Fig. 2).

Endoscopic Findings

In all 213 patients who underwent endoscopy, worms were removed by biopsy forceps (Fig. 3), and a definite diagnosis of anisakiasis was made. The *Anisakis* worms were present in all areas of the mucosal surface of the stomach. A diagram of the stomach was made by theoretically opening the stomach along the greater curvature. The actual sites of infiltrating larvae were then accurately mapped. While the larvae infested all areas of the stomach, they were densely distributed in the corpus and along the angle.

Fig. 4. Endoscopic findings of tumor-formation type

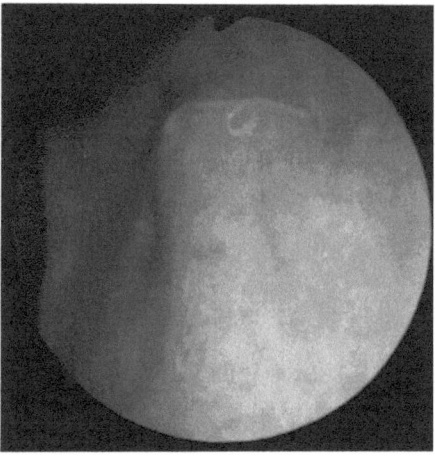

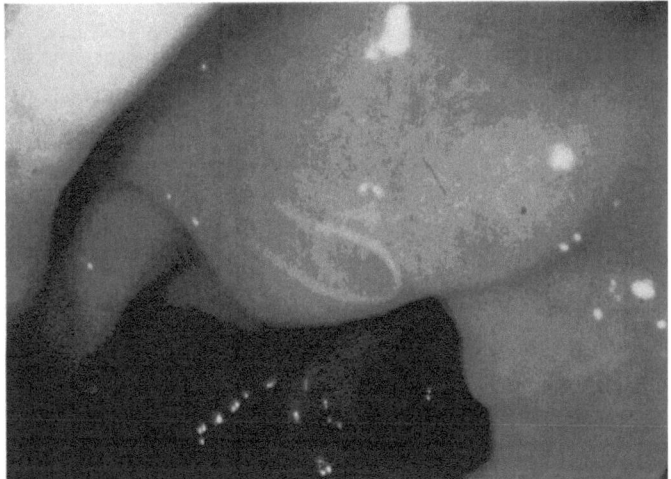

Fig. 5. Endoscopic findings of swollen-fold type

Findings at site of infestation. The local findings of the infestation sites of *Anisakis* larva were classified into the following three types: (a) Tumor-formation type—entrance at the center of an elevation with an ill-defined border (Fig. 4); (b) swollen-fold type—entrance through the top or bottom of an edematous mucosal fold (Fig. 5); (c) flat and no-change type—entrance into a flat mucosa with an elevation of neither the mucosa nor edematous folds (Fig. 3).

Using this classification, the flat type was seen in 34 (16.0%), the tumor-formation type in 92 (43.2%), and the swollen-fold type in 87 patients (40.8%; Table 2).

At the actual site of infestation, a mild spotty hemorrhage or a mild erosion was seen in 55 patients (Fig. 6).

Table 2. Endoscopic findings in 213 patients

	No. of cases	Percent
Local findings at site of infestation		
Flat and no change	34	16.0
Tumor formation	92	43.2
Swelling of folds	87	40.8
Edema		
Absent	31	14.6
Present		
Partial	82	38.5
Widespread		
Slight	73	34.3
Extensive	27	12.7

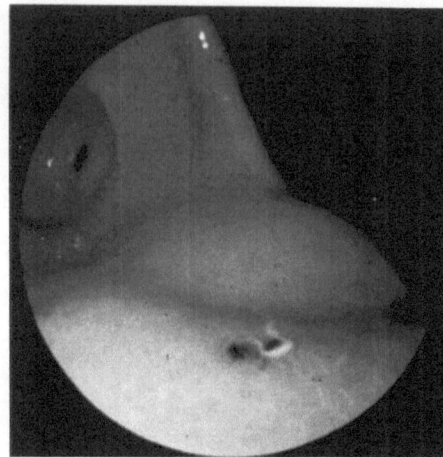

Fig. 6. Endoscopic findings. A mild spotty hemorrhage is seen at the site of infestation

Mucosal findings away from site of infestation. Diffuse mucosal edema was usually noted in addition to the above-described findings at the entrance site (Fig. 7). This edema was then classified into four types: (a) A practical absence of edema in the entire stomach was seen in 31 patients (14.6%). (b) Partial edema in part of the stomach was seen in 82 patients (38.5%). (c) Slightly widespread edema, which covered almost the entire mucosal surface of the stomach, was present in 73 patients (34.3%). (d) Extensive widespread edema, which was diffuse and caused an actual narrowing of the lumen, was noted in 27 patients (12.7%; Fig. 7).

In many patients, there were changes in the gastric mucosa which were not directly related to the larvae. Such changes as severe erosion, spotty hemorrhage (Fig. 7), and ulcers were also observed.

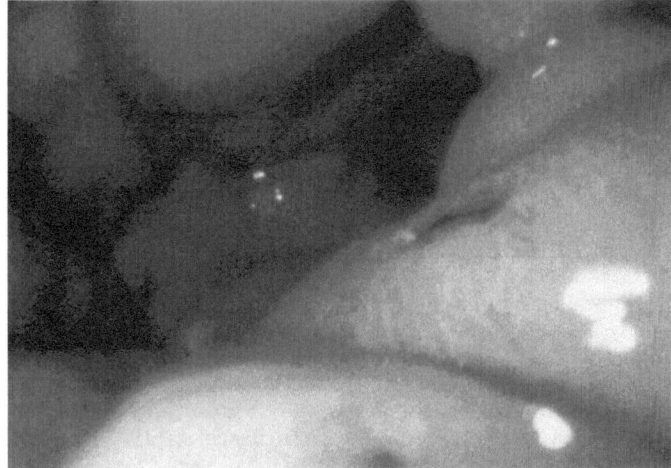

Fig. 7. Endoscopic findings. Widespread edema is seen over the entire stomach. A spotty hemorrhage, also present in the mucosa, is not directly affected by the larvae

Discussion

Acute gastric anisakiasis is characterized by a sudden onset of violent gastric pain. A laparotomy is at times performed under the diagnosis of an acute abdomen [1]. *Anisakis* infestation should always be considered in patients with violent epigastric pain and particularly when it is known that the patient has eaten raw mackerel. Other common symptoms are nausea, anorexia, and vomitting, which are also characteristic of acute gastritis [2–5]. Since the larvae of *Anisakis* can consistently be observed endoscopically, early endoscopy is highly recommended for patients in whom acute gastric anisakiasis is suspected and for those who have eaten raw fish within 12 h before the onset of gastric symptoms. In some cases, symptoms are similar to those of gastric anisakiasis, however no larva of *Anisakis* can be detected in the stomach. In such cases, we would suspect intestinal anisakiasis.

It should be emphasized that the mucosal changes in acute gastric anisakiasis are not confined to the site of penetration alone but are also present in other areas. The local reaction of the mucosa where the larvae penetrate is generally mild with a slight elevation or swelling of the folds. Even in 16% of the patients we examined, the actual site of entrance was flat with no discernible change. Spotty hemorrhage or erosion was locally seen at the site of penetration in only 25.8% of 213 patients. The most characteristic mucosal change was edema of a variable degree, ranging from zero or mild to an extensive spread. This mucosal edema, identifiable using an endoscope or in barium studies, may be produced histologically by the edema not only in the tunica mucosa but also in both the tunica mucosa and tela submucosa. This edema rapidly disappears after removal of the larvae. Many cases of acute gastric anisakiasis belong to the edematous type according to our classification of acute gastritis [5].

We have clinically experienced gastric edema in the absence of *Anisakis* infestation, and in about 10% of patients with gastric anisakiasis, no gastric edema was exhibited. However, in the majority of patients with acute gastritis of the edematous type, anisakiasis should be suspected.

References

1. Ishikura H (1969) Occurrence of anisakiasis and its clinical presentation. Saishin Igaku 24: 357–365 (in Japanese)
2. Sugimachi K, Inokuchi K, Ooiwa T, Fujino T, Ishii Y (1985) Acute gastric anisakiasis. Analysis of 178 cases. JAMA 253: 1012–1013
3. Fujino T, Ooiwa T, Ishii Y (1984) Clinical, epidemiological and morphological studies on 150 cases of acute gastric anisakiasis in Fukuoka prefecture. Jpn J Parasitol 33: 73–92 (English abstract)
4. Matsukuma A, Mori M, Ooiwa T, Sugimachi K (1987) Vanishing tumor of the stomach. Am J Gastroenterol 82: 1102–1103
5. Sugimachi K, Inokuchi K, Kuwano H, Ooiwa T (1984) Acute gastritis clinically classified in accordance with data from both upper GI series and endoscopy. Scand J Gastroenterol 19: 31–37

Radiographic Examination

T. KUSUHARA and M. FUKUDA

A major cause of infection by *Anisakis* larvae is the eating of uncooked fish. Accordingly gastric anisakis is common in Japan, where raw fish is frequently consumed.

Gastric anisakiasis has two forms—acute and chronic. Both types are caused by an infection of *Anisakis* larvae. The acute or fulminant type of gastric anisakiasis is commonly encountered. This type may occur as a result of allergic reactions induced by secondary infection [1]. The most common symptom is upper abdominal cramps, which occur several hours after eating uncooked fish infected with *Anisakis*. The term "acute gastric anisakiasis" was first introduced by Namiki et al. [2], who demonstrated radiographically an *Anisakis* larva in the stomach and successfully removed it using the endoscopic technique. An *Anisakis* larva is seen radiographically as a linear translucency of various shapes with gastric mucosal edema on double-contrast images [3].

Nakata et al. [4] emphasized that the most important radiological finding was the demonstration of a threadlike filling defect; suggestive but indeterminate findings, such as coarse, broad gastric folds due to mucosal edema, were also evident. In no case was the radiological examination negative. The worm was detected in 76% of cases (31/41) in their study.

Shibata et al. [5] analyzed the gastric X-ray findings in relation to the site of penetration into the gastric wall in 100 cases of acute gastric anisakiasis. Characteristic findings were poor adhesion of barium to the gastric mucosa, spreading of the gastric angle, abnormalities of both the greater and lesser curvature lines, and edematous hypertrophic folds. Spreading of the gastric angle could be clearly observed in all cases with penetration at the region near the gastric angle and in many cases with penetration at the cardiac region. Both gastric curvature lines showed straightening and irregularity, and these abnormal findings were more frequently seen in the cases with penetration on the greater curvature side than on the other side. Those abnormalities were evident on the anal side with respect to the point of penetration. The edematous hypertrophic folds were parallel to the gastric axis, and the long folds were found in the cases with penetration at the proximal gastric region and the greater curvature side. It may be concluded that inflammation of the gastric mucosa as a result of penetration extends in an anal direction from the penetration point. The detectability of a worm was 60% (60/100) in their report [5].

Yoh and Tsushimi [6] recorded that X-ray examinations revealed the marginal rigidity of the gastric outline, which was marked by a swelling of the mucosa and a wider gastric angle, and that these findings were similar to those in gastric allergies.

Fujino et al. [7] classified the invasion of the gastric mucosa in 113 cases into three types: a simple elevation of the mucosa (tumor-formation type); a swollen or infolded mucosal membrane (swelling of fold type); and a flat mucosal surface with a normal form (normal type). However, varying degrees of edema were apparent on the gastric wall in most cases; the appearance was normal in other cases. They noted that severe cases of edema in anisakiasis fall into the category of the edematous type in the classification of acute gastritis. The tumor-formation type in their classification may be the so-called vanishing tumor of the stomach [8]. Characteristic features of the vanishing tumor are a fulminant occurrence and rapid regression of the local lesion; the tumor may also show localized edema with acute gastritis or an accumulation of serous fluid under the mucosal membrane [9]. An acquired factor (allergy, drug, or parasite) is thought to be the cause of the vanishing tumor [10]. There are reports suggesting a connection between the vanishing tumor and *Anisakis* larvae [11–14], and the worm has been observed on the surface of the tumor [15–17].

In the study by Sugimachi et al. [18], threadlike filling defects approximately 30 mm in length, were characteristic of the disease and were found in 62 of 130 patients who underwent an upper gastrointestinal (GI) tract series. The defect was usually circular, though the shape was occasionally different. An adequate compression technique as well as double-contrast study are useful in identification of the worms. Mucosal edema was usually present (80.8%). Mucosal edema was visualized radiographically as a broad gastric fold with or without widening of the gastric angle. These findings are not definitive, but in an appropriate clinical setting, they are highly suggestive of anisakiasis. The diagnosis was confirmed endoscopically in the cases where a worm was not detected in the radiographic examination. The differential diagnosis from gastric tumor or cancer is essential because of mucosal changes; endoscopy has proved to be a far more effective approach for a correct diagnosis.

In our investigation [19, 20] of 226 patients, gastric mucosal edema, radiographically defined as coarse and broad gastric folds with or without widening of the gastric angle (Figs. 1, 2), was seen in 224 cases (98%). In 179 cases (88%), the mucosal edema was so extensive that it occupied more than half of the entire gastric wall (Fig. 3). Localized swelling of the gastric mucosa was sometimes manifest on the radiograph as a vanishing tumor (Fig. 4). The gastric wall usually appeared soft and with good extensibility, though the mucosal changes caused by extensive edema frequently resembled those seen in Borrmann's type IV advanced gastric cancer (Fig. 5). The radiographic diagnosis of acute gastric anisakiasis was most often observed when a threadlike filling defect caused by the presence of an *Anisakis* larva was seen in the area of mucosal edema. The filling defect was usually 3 cm in length and straight, serpentine, or circular (Figs. 6, 7). This was radiographically observed in 139 cases (61%).

Nagano et al. [21] and Doi [22] think that this type of acute gastric anisakiasis occurs not only as a result of *Anisakis* larvae but also *Terranova* larvae. Cases with *Terranova* larvae have mostly been reported in the north of Japan (especial-

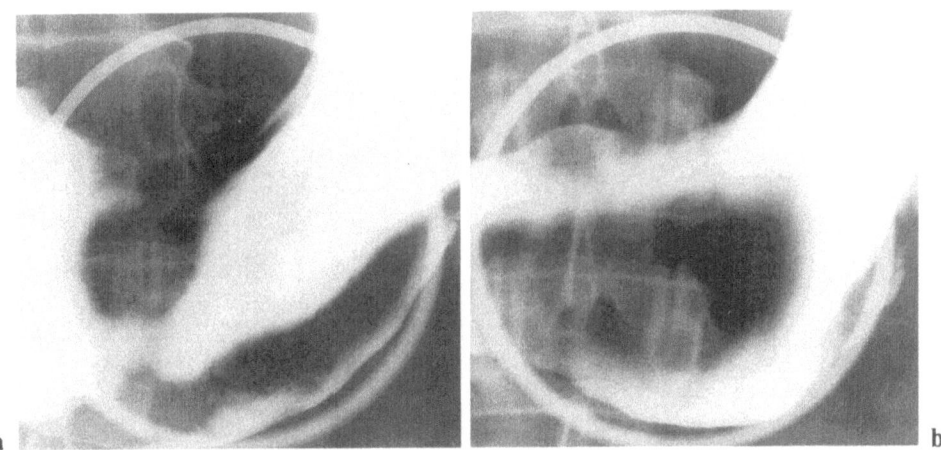

Fig. 1a, b. Typical features of the mucosal edema are shown as coarse and broad mucosal folds in a compression study

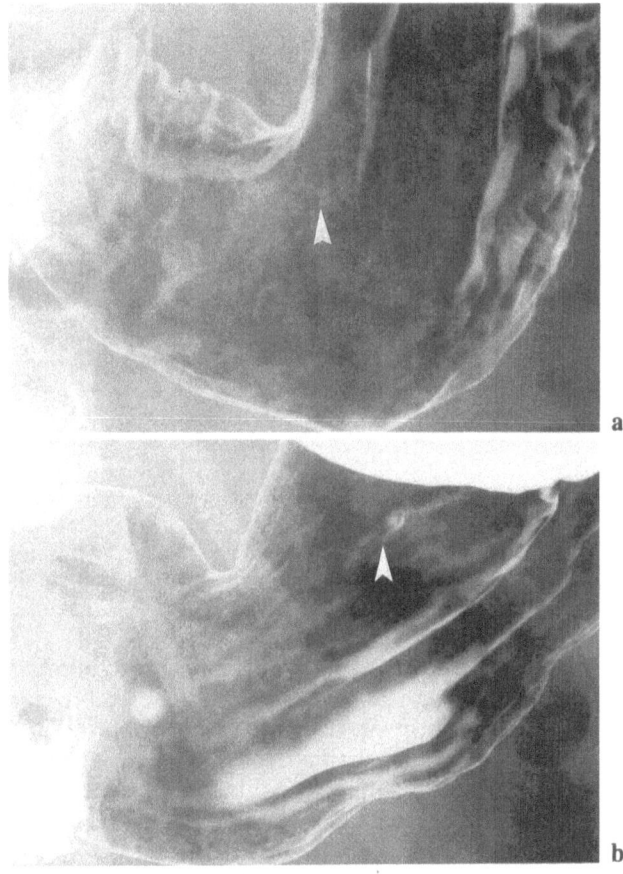

Fig. 2a, b. Mucosal edema extends **a** with and **b** without widening of the gastric angle in a double-contrast study. *Arrows* show *Anisakis* worms

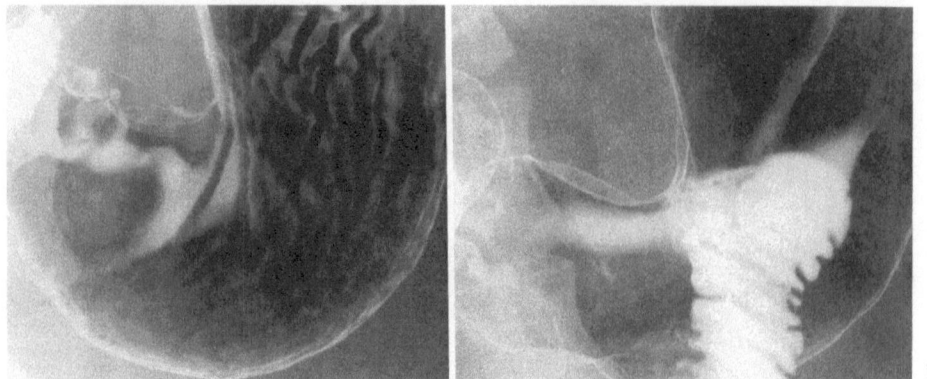

a   b

Fig. 3a, b. The spread of mucosal edema appears **a** over half of the gastric antrum and angle and **b** over three-quarters of the gastric wall from the gastric antrum to the body

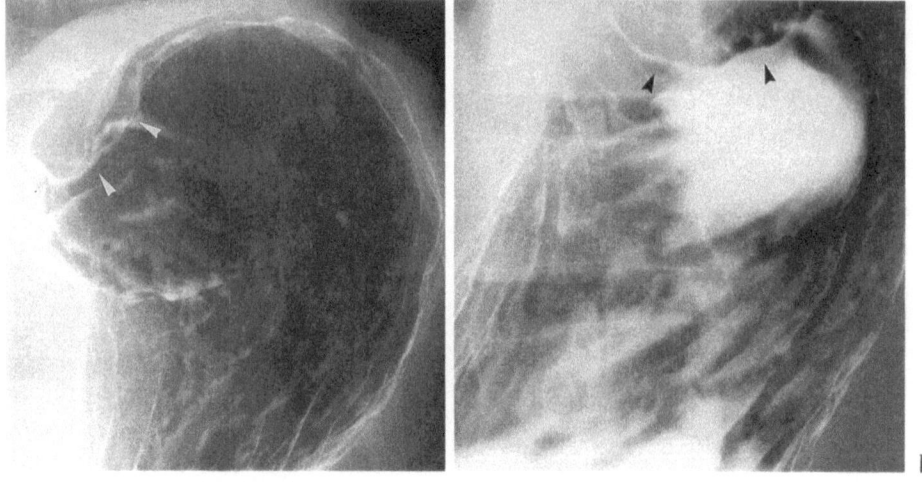

a   b

Fig. 4a, b. A tumor-like shadow (so-called vanishing tumor) is shown at the gastric fornix. **a** Upright position; **b** double-contrast study in the left anterior oblique position

ly Hokkaido), but there have been no reports from the south. The reason why the incidence of this disease is observed to vary geographically may be due to differences in the geographical distribution of fish species and the final host of the two types of larva. Doi [22] describes that an *Anisakis* larva is seen radiographically as a thin threadlike radiolucency; a *Terranova* larva, on other hand, is visualized as a thicker, stringlike radiolucency in double-contrast or compression images, and differentiation between the two is not so difficult. However, Doi says that the two kinds of worm do not show any difference radiographically on the gastric mucosa, such as dilatation of the gastric angle or swollen mucosal folds, which would provide a most important clue toward identification.

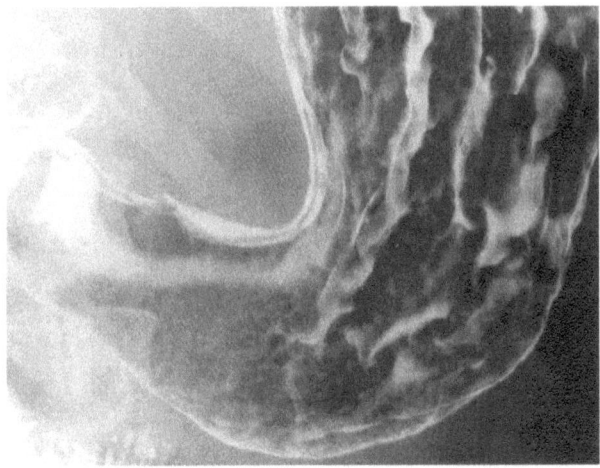

Fig. 5. The marginal rigidity on the lesser curvature of the gastric antrum and mucosal changes caused by extensive edema, resembling those seen in Borrmann's type IV of advanced gastric cancer

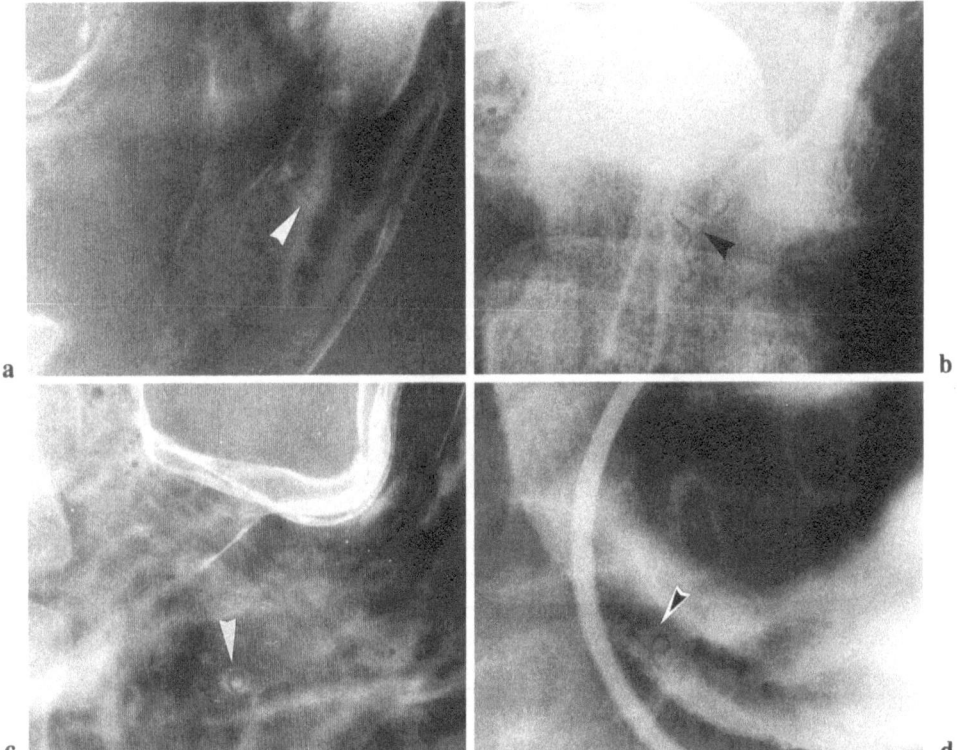

Fig. 6a–d. Typical threadlike filling defects caused by *Anisakis* larvae are shown as **a** straight, **b** serpentine, **c** circular, and **d** double ring-like

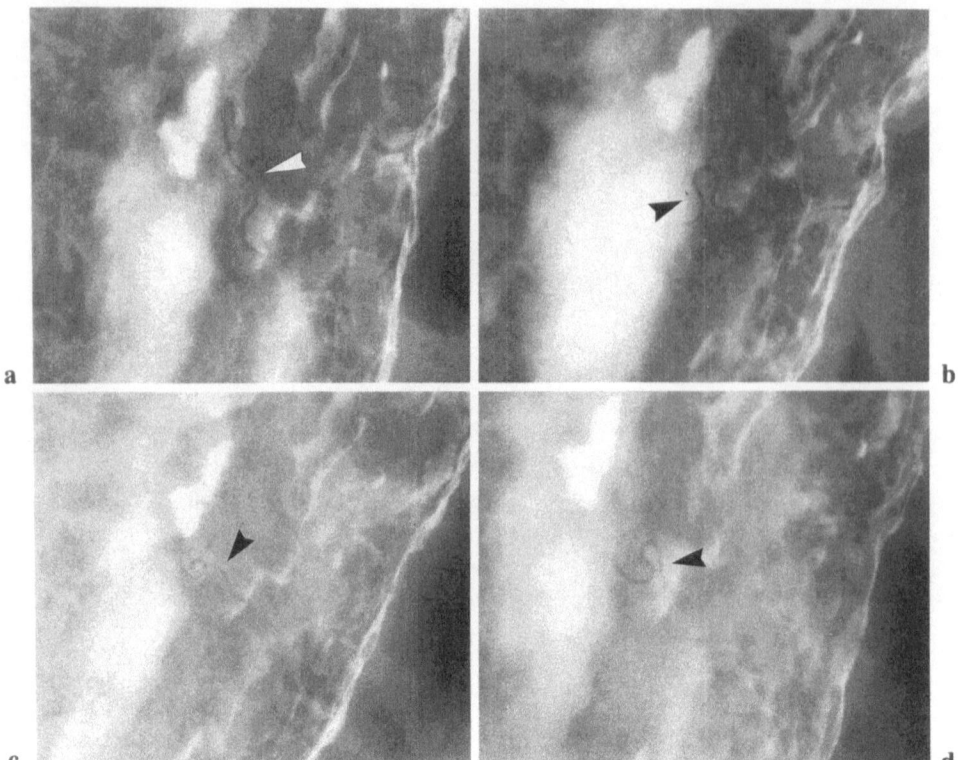

Fig. 7a–d. The shape of a threadlike filling defect changes during examination of UGI upper gastrointestinal tract series

In conclusion, the acute or fulminant type of gastric anisakiasis may occur as a result of allergic reactions induced by the secondary infection. Therefore, on radiographic examination, this disease usually appears as the edematous type of acute gastritis [23], which is allergic gastritis of acute gastric mucosal lesions. Mucosal edema, which can be seen over an extensive area as coarse, broad gastric folds, is the basic radiographic finding of this disease. This finding is not definitive, but it is highly suggestive of acute gastric anisakiasis in a patient with an appropriate clinical history. In almost all cases, upper GI tract series commonly show that a rapid disappearance of mucosal edema occurs during the first 1–2 weeks. The most definitive diagnostic radiographic finding is the appearance of a threadlike filling defect in the area of the mucosal edema. This filling defect reveals the *Anisakis* larva itself and is evident at the greater curvature from the gastric antrum to the body in many cases.

The detectability of a worm on radiographic examination is less frequent than on endoscopic examination, and there are the demerits of X-ray exposure to be considered with the former. Therefore, we think endoscopic examination should be adopted as the preferable method in the diagnosis and treatment of acute gastric anisakiasis.

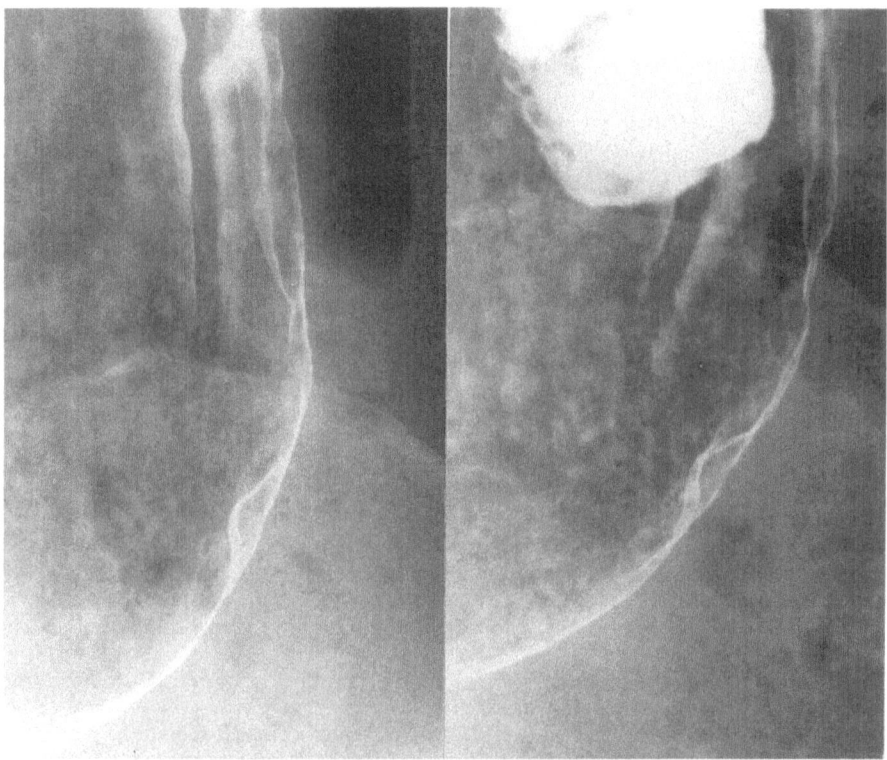

Fig. 8. Eosinophilic granuloma due to *Anisakis* larva are shown as an elevated lesion which looks like a submucosal tumor

The chronic type may be due to primary infection by an *Anisakis* larva [1]. In this type, a granuloma forms, the core of which is a worm. The granuloma develops in the submucosal layer at the point where the larva penetrated the tissue; this type is, therefore, termed parasitic eosinophilic granuloma. This disease is usually discovered during a diagnostic course for other GI symptoms or diseases some time after the original infection, because the symptoms are mild or negative.

The radiographic findings here are similar to those of a submucosal tumor or type IIa + IIc of early gastric cancer; a detailed description of these findings is thus omitted in the present chapter. Parasitic eosinophilic granuloma is a rare disease, and radiographically it has no distinctive findings. Therefore, this disease may be diagnosed commonly as the former two diseases by radiographic examination. Consequently, endoscopic examination (dye test or biopsy) is necessary for a definitive diagnosis of the chronic type. The correct diagnosis can be confirmed by pathological examination of a resected specimen. Figure 8 shows the radiographic features of an eosinophilic granuloma caused by an *Anisakis* larva.

References

1. Miyazato T (1980) Studies on the eosinophilic granuloma formation in parasitic infections with special reference to the experimental gastric anisakiasis. Med J Kinki Univ 5: 157–180 (in Japanese)
2. Namiki T, Morooka T, Kawauchi H, Ueda N, Sekiya C, Nakagawa K, Furuta T, Oguro T, Kamata H (1970) Diagnosis of acute gastric anisakiasis. Stomach Intestine 5: 1437–1440 (in Japanese)
3. Kawauchi H, Nmiki T, Morooka T, Nakagawa K, Oguro T (1973) Gastric anisakiasis presenting acute gastrointestinal symptoms—with special references to the endoscopic and roentgenographic findings of anisakis larva penetrating into the wall of the human stomach and to its clinical features. Stomach Intestine 8: 31–38 (in Japanese)
4. Nakata H, Takeda K, Nakayama T (1980) Radiological diagnosis of acute gastric anisakiasis. Radiology 135: 49–53
5. Shibata O, Ichimanda M, Furusawa T, Arita T, Kudou T, Emoto O (1981) Investigation of acute gastric anisakiasis—especially on findings of the x-ray examination of the stomach. Nagasaki Med J 56: 20–25 (in Japanese)
6. Yoh T, Tsushimi K (1981) Acute gastric anisakiasis—with special references to clinical features and its roentgenological and endoscopic findings. Arch Jpn Chir 50: 229–234 (in Japanese)
7. Fujino T, Oiwa T, Isii Y (1984) Clinical, epidemilogical and morphological studies on 150 cases of acute gastric anisakiasis in Fukuoka prefecture. Jpn J Parasitol 33: 73–92 (in Japanese)
8. Yamasaki M (1976) Vanishing tumor of the stomach? Jpn J Clin Radiol 21: 47–54 (in Japanese)
9. Yamasaki M, Hara K, Shinbo T (1978) On the vanishing tumor of the stomach (the second report). Jpn J Clin Radiol 23: 919–924 (in Japanese)
10. Okazaki Y, Azuma M, Kawahara K, Hirata M, Nakamura K, Takemoto T, Eguchi S (1978) A case of so-called vanishing tumor of the stomach accompanied with small ulcer endoscopically. Jpn J Gastroenterol 75: 902–908 (in Japanese)
11. Toda M, Okazaki Y, Azuma M, Maetani N, Saito M, Odawara M, Fujita K, Harima T, Ariyama S, Miyazaki S, Harada H, Iida Y, Kawamura S, Takemoto T, Urayama S (1980) A case of acute gastritis resembling process of vanishing tumor. Gastroenterol Endoscopy 22: 1085–1090 (in Japanese)
12. Yokoya H, Ooe K, Miyoshi S, Hidaka T, Murakami Y, Tsuji M (1980) Three cases of acute gastric anisakiasis—especially of its seroimmunological diagnosis. Stomach Intestine 15: 1329–1335 (in Japanese)
13. Kinoshita Z, Kinoshita K, Hino K, Nishimura S, Numa Y, Maetani N, Odawara M, Shimizu M, Iida Y, Hamada Y, Tada M, Kawashima M, Takemoto T (1984) Two cases of acute gastric lesion assuming the form of gastric vanishing tumor. Gastroenterol Endoscopy 26: 884–887 (in Japanese)
14. Muraoka H, Suzuki S, Okuaki K, Azuma K, Kimura K (1984) A case of "vanishing tumor of the stomach" due to parasitosis. Gastroenterol Endoscopy 26: 1719–1724 (in Japanese)
15. Shinoshima F, Yamasaki H, Kawauchi H, Hirao M, Sato F (1980) Vanishing tumor of the stomach (?), report of two cases. Med J Hokkaido Ass Med Med Surv Workers 7: 40–44 (in Japanese)
16. Mikami Y (1983) The submucosal tumor due to anisakis larva at the fornix of the stomach. Shimane Med 6: 871–877 (in Japanese)
17. Hirota K, Uchida Y, Hatano Y, Yasutake R, Okazaki Y, Takemoto T, Fujii Y, Iwata T (1986) A case of gastric anisakiasis taking the course of vanishing tumor of the stomach. Gastoenterol Endoscopy 28: 789–794 (in Japanese)
18. Sugimachi K, Inokuchi K, Oiwa T, Fujino T, Ishii Y (1985) Acute gastric anisakiasis-analysis of 178 cases. JAMA 253: 1012–1013

19. Kusuhara T (1983) Clinical study of acute gastric anisakiasis: II. Radiological and endoscopical features. J Kumamoto Med Soc 57: 69–79 (in Japanese)
20. Kusuhara T, Watanabe K, Fukuda M (1984) Radiographic study of acute gastric anisakiasis. Gastrointest Radiol 9: 305–309
21. Nagano K, Takagi K, Yanagawa K, Oishi K, Kagei N (1973) Acute heterocheilidiasis of the stomach (due to *Terranova decipiens*). Stomach Intestine 8: 81–85 (in Japanese)
22. Doi K (1973) Clinical aspects of acute heterrocheilidiasis of the stomach (due to the larvae of *Anisakis* and *Terranova decipiens*)—especially on its differential diagnosis by x-ray and endoscopy. Stomach Intestine 8: 1513–1518 (in Japanese)
23. Oiwa T (1973) A clinical study of acute gastritis. Stomach Intestine 8: 1223–1230 (in Japanese)

Ultrasonic Examination

M. Yano, S. Yokomizo, and T. Nakayama

Introduction

The diagnosis of gastric diseases by ultrasonography has been considered to be relatively difficult because of the presence of digestive tract gas, which is most disadvantageous for ultrasonography, and the thickness of the organ, which is several millimeters thick. However, with improvements in ultrasonographic diagnostic equipment, many reports have appeared recently showing its applicability in the diagnosis of gastric diseases, such as gastric cancer, gastritis, and gastric ulcer [1–3]. Gastric anisakiasis causes such symptoms as severe epigastric pain, but if the larva is extracted endoscopically the symptoms disappear rapidly [4]. An early diagnosis is important in this disease. Gastric anisakiasis can be diagnosed by ultrasonography as a thickening of the gastric wall, and this is very useful as a supplementary means of diagnosis to endoscopy. In this chapter, ultrasonography of gastric anisakiasis is described mainly on the basis of the cases experienced by the authors.

Subjects and Methods

The subjects consisted of seven cases of gastric anisakiasis, in which we performed ultrasonography over a period of 3 years and 7 months from January 1983 to July 1986. Confirmatory diagnosis was made in six cases by endoscopic identification of the larva and in one case by roentgenological visualization of the larva. In these cases, ultrasonography was performed prior to roentgenography or endoscopy of the stomach.

All the patients complained chiefly of epigastric pain, and no special measures, such as the gastric filling method with drinking water, were taken except in one case in which fasting only was practised before the examination. The method of scanning was both longitudinal and transverse over the region of the stomach, and other organs in the abdominal cavity, such as the liver, gallbladder, and pancreas, were examined simultaneously.

The equipment used included linear electron scanners, Aloka SSD 250, 256, and Toshiba SAL-90A, Japan.

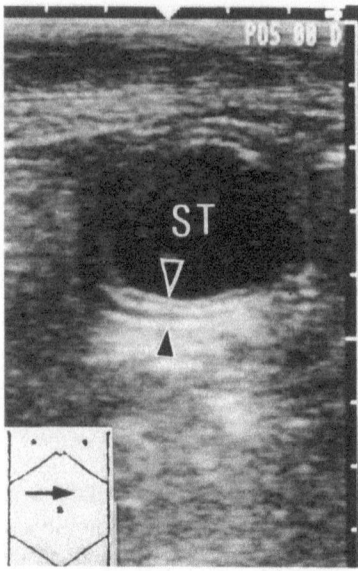

Fig. 1. Normal ultrasonogram of the stomach wall (arrow)

Ultrasonogram of Normal Stomach

The thickness of the normal gastric wall is less than 5 mm [5], and it presents a five-layer structure under current ultrasonographic diagnostic equipment with high image resolution. The order is as follows: high-echo zone, low-echo zone, high-echo zone, low-echo zone, and high-echo zone [6]. Figure 1 shows a normal ultrasonogram of the stomach.

Ultrasonogram of Gastric Anisakiasis

Table 1 shows the findings by ultrasonography, gastric endoscopy, and gastric roentgenography in seven patients who visited our clinic. An image of gastric wall thickening was seen in all of the seven cases in the echo findings, five cases showing a generalized thickening and two localized thickening. No stratified structures were noted in the thickened part of the wall in any of the cases, and an image with a uniform low echo was evident. In addition, the thickened part of the wall in two cases presenting a localized wall thickening image in the echo was in good agreement with the lesioned part observed by gastric endoscopy, which was performed after echo examination. In six of seven cases, the larva was extracted endoscopically with biopsy forceps, and the symptoms then improved rapidly. One patient refused endoscopy, and the treatment was conducted by means of drugs.

   In cases 1 and 2, an abdominal echo was performed 1 month after extraction of the larva, and it revealed complete disappearance of the gastric wall thickening. In one case, 300 ml water was consumed by the patient at the time of the echo examination, and the extensibility of the thickened wall was observed.

Table 1. Patient findings with gastric anisakiasis

Case no.	Age (yrs)	Sex	Ultrasound	Gastric endoscopy	Gastric X-ray	Prognosis
1	20	F	Generalized thickening of gastric wall (15 mm)	Redness, erosion, and *Anisakis* body on greater curvature in upper part of gastric body	Not performed	Rapid improvement after extraction of larva with gastric endoscopy
2	42	M	Generalized thickening of gastric wall (15 mm)	Redness, edema, shadow ulcer, and *Anisakis* body on greater curvature in upper part of gastric body	Not performed	Rapid improvement after extraction of larva with gastric endoscopy
3	49	M	Generalized thickening of gastric wall (15 mm)	Not performed	Edema and *Anisakis* body on anterior wall of gastric body	Treatment with medication alone
4	44	M	Generalized thickening of gastric wall (20 mm)	Redness, edema, and *Anisakis* body on posterior wall in upper part of gastric body	Not performed	Rapid improvement after extraction of larva with gastric endoscopy
5	28	M	Generalized thickening of gastric wall (15 mm)	Redness, edema, and *Anisakis* body on greater curvature of lower part of gastric body	Performed after extraction of larva with gastric endoscopy; edema in lower part of gastric body	Rapid improvement after extraction of larva with gastric endoscopy
6	29	M	Localized thickening of anterior wall of gastric body (11 mm)	Edema and *Anisakis* body on anterior wall of gastric body	Not performed	Rapid improvement after extraction of larva with gastric endoscopy
7	44	F	Localized thickening of posterior wall of gastric body (10 mm)	*Anisakis* body in posterior wall in middle part of gastric body	Image of parasite on posterior wall in middle part of gastric body	Rapid improvement after extraction of larva with gastric endoscopy

Concerning the ultrasonographic diagnosis of gastric anisakiasis, Iizuka and Maki [7] reported two cases, stating that both presented an image of gastric wall thickening around the entire circumference; the surface was smooth, the inside consisted of a uniform echo, not separable into single layers, and extensibility of the thickened wall was observed in one case after drinking water. Ogata et al. [8] reported two cases, stating that a characteristic finding is localized gastric wall thickening and the influence of peristaltic movement. We experienced five cases of generalized thickening and two cases of localized thickening, and it would seem that two types of wall thickening images occur. Further, Iizuka and Maki [7] state that ultrasonography is useful for judging the healing of gastric anisa-kiasis, as the echo in the abdominal region 1 month after extraction of the larva revealed disappearance of the gastric wall thickening. We have also noted the disappearance of gastric wall thickening in an echo performed 1 month after extraction of the larva, and it seems that ultrasonography is useful for assessing the healing of gastric anisakiasis.

Case Reports

Case 1

The patient was a 20-year-old female whose chief complaint was epigastralgia. On the evening of 30 January 1983, the subject ate raw mackerel. Eight hours later, nausea, vomiting, and epigastralgia occurred, and the subject was admitted to our hospital.

Abdominal ultrasonic findings. The gastric wall evidently swelled to a thickness of about 15 mm (Fig. 2). Since gastric anisakiasis was suspected from the symptoms and echo findings, the stomach was immediately examined endoscopically.

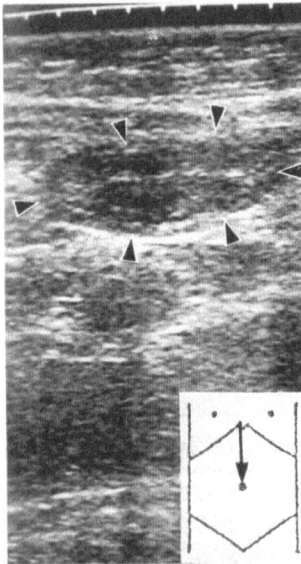

Fig. 2. Abdominal ultrasound. The gastric wall evidently swelled to a thickness of about 15 mm (arrow)

Fig. 3. Gastric endoscopy. In the greater curvature of the upper part, rubor and erosion were noted. A larva of Anisakis was found in the area

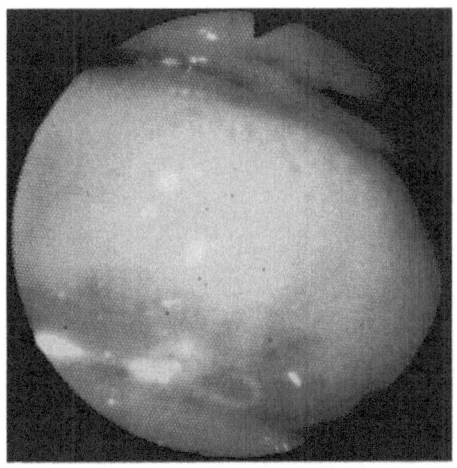

Fig. 4. Abdominal echo image taken 1 month later. The gastric wall (arrow) had shrunk to the normal thickness of 4 mm

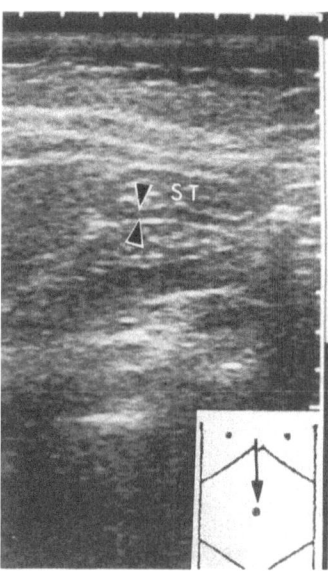

Gastric endoscopic findings. In the greater curvature of the upper part, rubor and erosion were noted. A larva of *Anisakis* was found in the area (Fig. 3) and removed by forceps.

After removal, the pain subsided quickly. Figure 4 is an abdominal echo image taken 1 month later, and the gastric wall had shrunk to the normal thickness of 4 mm.

Case 2

The patient was a 44-year-old male whose chief complaint was epigastralgia. On the evening of 8 February 1986, the patient ate a raw sardine. Epigastralgia

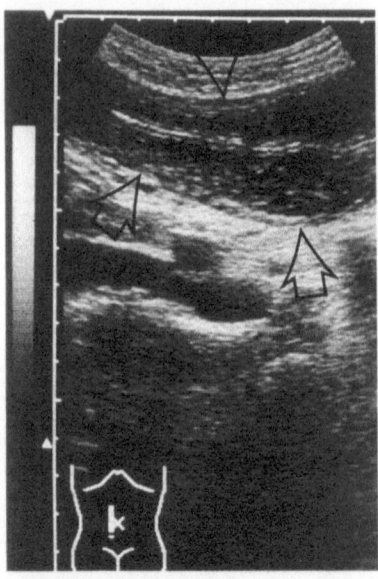

Fig. 5. Abdominal ultrasound. The gastric wall (arrow) was completely swollen to a thickness of about 20 mm

began on the evening of the next day, and the pain had not subsided by 10 February when the subject was admitted to our hospital. After examination, the abdominal echo picture was taken.

Abdominal ultrasonic findings. The gastric wall was completely swollen to a thickness of about 20 mm (Fig. 5). A gastric fiberscope was then applied.

Gastric endoscopic findings. Rubor and edema were noted in the posterior wall of the upper part of the stomach, and a worm was found in the area. It was removed using bioassay forceps.

Case 3

The patient was a 44-year-old female whose chief complaint was epigastric pain. On the evening of 23 July 1986, the patient ate raw horse-mackerel. At about 2 a.m., epigastric pain started, which did not subside, and the patient was admitted to our hospital
    Ultrasonography in the abdominal region was performed immediately after the physical examination. The posterior wall of the gastric body showed localized thickening to about 10 mm, but the anterior wall showed no thickening, and it seemed that only the posterior wall had localized thickening (Fig. 6).

Contrast roentgenography of the upper digestive tract. In gastric X-ray performed after the echo of the abdominal region, a linear shadow was noted on the posterior wall in the middle part of the gastric body, which seemed to be the body of an *Anisakis* larva (Fig. 7). Gastric endoscopy was performed the next day. A parasite was noted on the posterior wall in the middle part of the gastric

Fig. 6. Ultrasonography in
the abdominal region. The
posterior wall of the gastric
body (large arrow) showed
localized thickening to
about 10 mm, but the
anterior wall (small arrow)
showed no thickening

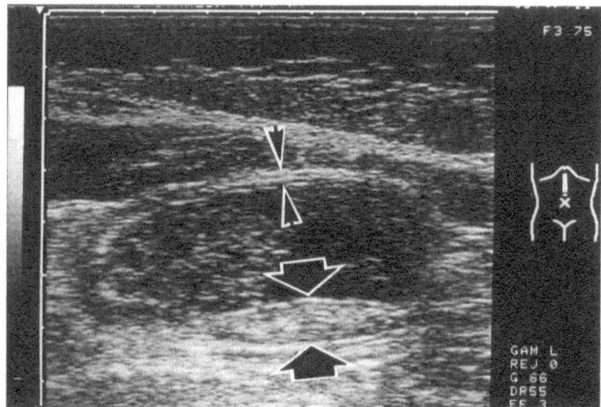

Fig. 7. Gastric X-ray. A linear shadow was
noted on the posterior wall in the middle part of
the gastric body, which seemed to be the body
of an Anisakis larva

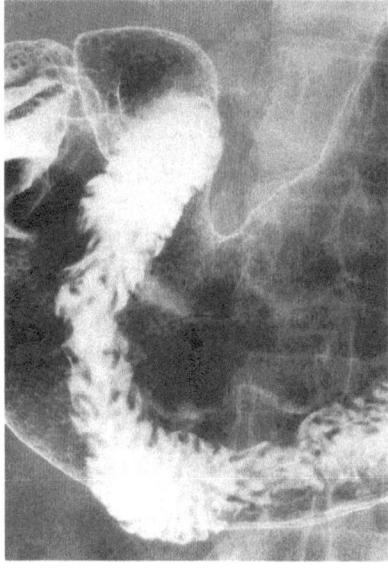

body, which was extracted with biopsy forceps. The parasite was identified as a
larva of the genus *Anisakis*.

After extraction of the larva, the symptoms disappeared immediately.

Differential Diagnosis from Other Gastric Diseases by Ultrasonography

Acute Gastritis

An image of the total circumferential wall thickening with an internal uniform
low echo is made. Extensibility of the gastric wall is maintained, and it is difficult
to differentiate this condition from gastric anisakiasis presenting total circum-

ferential wall thickening. However, differentiation is possible in most cases if the anamnesis is taken into consideration.

Gastric Ulcer

In the case of deep and large ulcers, the localized wall thickening is visualized with the low-echo, high-echo part, which represents the ulcer. A problem is posed in differentiating gastric anisakiasis that shows a localized wall thickening image, but it seems that the high-echo part of the ulcer is not visualized in gastric anisakiasis.

Gastric Cancer

An image of gastric wall thickening is noted, reflecting the tumorous part, but the thicknesses of the swollen image and the internal echo are often not uniform. There is little extensibility of the thickened part, and it is easy to differentiate this condition from gastric anisakiasis.

Summary

The characteristic feature of an ultrasonogram in gastric anisakiasis is an image of low-echo wall thickening, and there are two types noted—total circumferential wall thickening and localized wall thickening. Extensibility was noted in the wall thickening after drinking water. The gastric wall recovered to a normal echo after extraction of the larva, and it seems that ultrasonography is useful for assessing the healing of anisakiasis.

References

1. Walls WJ (1976) The evaluation of malignant gastric neoplasms by ultrasound B-scanning. Radiology 118: 159–163
2. Rosenberg ER, Morgan CL, Trought WS, Oddson TA (1980) The ultrasonic recognition of a gastric ulcer. Br J Radiol 53: 1014–1016
3. Asai H, Ogata K, Ichiyoshi M, Tanaka K (1981) Ultrasonographic approach to gastric diseases. Jpn J Med Ultrasonics 8: 237–243 (abstract in English)
4. Akasaka Y, Kizu M, Aoike A, Kawai K (1979) Endoscopic management of acute gastric anisakiasis. Endoscopy 2: 158–162
5. Karasawa E, Saotome N, Miki M, Ueno T (1980) Ultrasonography in gastrointestinal disease—ultrasonic evaluation of stomach wall. In: Proceedings of the 37th Meeting of the Japan Society of Ultrasonics in Medicine, Oct. 29, Yokohama, pp 399–400 (abstract in English)
6. Aibe T, Fuji T, Asagame F, Amano H, Kawashima M, Nagatomi Y, Harima K, Higashi M, Maetani N, Ariyama S, Goshima T, Kawamura S, Takemoto T (1982) The investigation of the ultrasonic endoscope, 2nd report. Gastroenterol Endoscopy 24: 1900–1909 (abstract in English)
7. Iizuka M, Maki T (1986) Diagnosis of gastric anisakiasis by ultrasonography. Nippon Rinshogeka Igakukai Zasshi 47: 100–104 (abstract in English)
8. Ogata K, Shimamoto H, Amako H, Asai H (1985) Ultrasonography of gastric anisakis. Proceedings of the 46th Meeting of the Japan Society of Ultrasonics in Medicine, June 29, Tokyo, pp 883–884 (abstract in English)

Contrast-Dye Method in Endoscopic Examination

Y. Hoshihara

Introduction

Namiki et al. [1] reported a case of acute gastric anisakiasis, in which so-called food poisoning symptoms appeared several hours after eating raw fish. Endoscopic examination revealed an *Anisakis*-like larva penetrating the gastric wall. Since then, many similar cases have been reported. Where the *Anisakis* larvae could be removed by biopsy forceps upon endoscopic examination, the symptoms subsequently disappeared. On the other hand, there are several cases [2] in which patients manifest the symptoms typical of acute gastric anisakiasis but lack evidence of an *Anisakis* larva upon endoscopic examination. In these cases, the contrast-dye method is very useful in demonstrating the larva to establish the diagnosis.

Contrast-Dye Method

We usually use the endoscopic contrast-dye method to make a differential diagnosis between benign gastric lesions and early gastric cancer [3, 4]. Through a sprayer inserted into the biopsy channel of the fiberscope, 0.1% indigo carmine solution is dispersed over the area of the lesion. Because this blue dye solution flows into the small concavities of the lesion, the slight undulations produce an excellent contrast. The irregularity can be detected and the pattern of the mucosal surface identified, which would not have been possible prior to application of the dye solution. We have experienced two cases [5] of anisakiasis without acute gastrointestinal symptoms, in which a larva was unexpectedly found by the contrast-dye method on endoscopic examination.

Cases

Case 1

This patient (72-year-old female) had no gastrointestinal symptoms such as abdominal pain, but the endoscopic examination was performed to search for

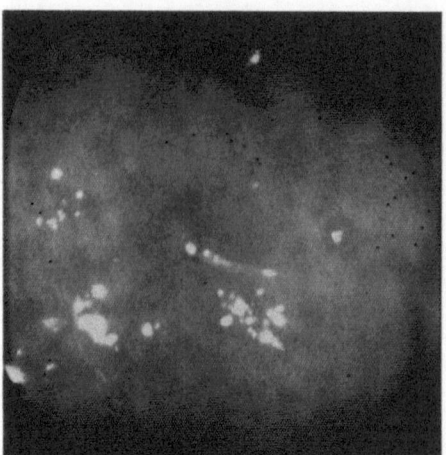

Fig. 1. A small elevated lesion observed by routine endoscopic examination. A larva is not evident

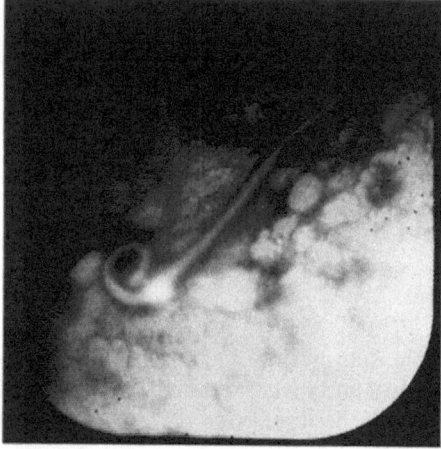

Fig. 2

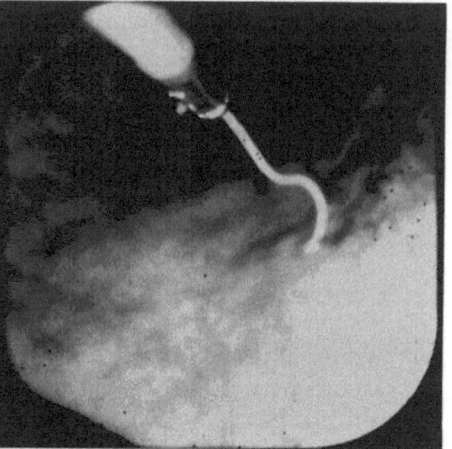

Fig. 3

Fig. 2. A slender larva penetrating the gastric wall demonstrated by means of the contrast-dye method on endoscopic examination

Fig. 3. A larva extracted by biopsy forceps on endoscopic examination

the cause of weight loss. We found only a small elevated lesion, about 2 mm in diameter, with a linear halation, about 5 mm in length, at the lesser curvature of the angulus of the stomach. This halation had the appearance of thread-like mucus (Fig. 1). By means of the contrast-dye method, however, we discovered a slender larva, about 2 cm in length, penetrating the elevated lesion (Fig. 2). The practical method for removing the larva by endoscopic biopsy forceps is shown in Fig. 3. Histological examination confirmed the identification as an *Anisakis* larva because a pair of bifoliate-like lateral chords were found in the cross section (Fig. 4).

Fig. 4. A cross section of the larva showing a pair of lateral chords and Y-shaped intestinal canal observed by histological examination

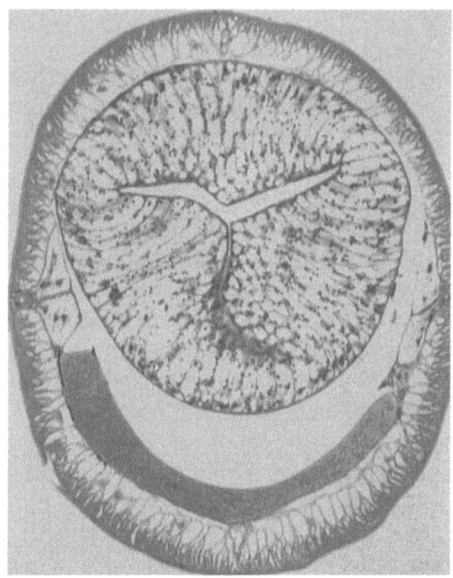

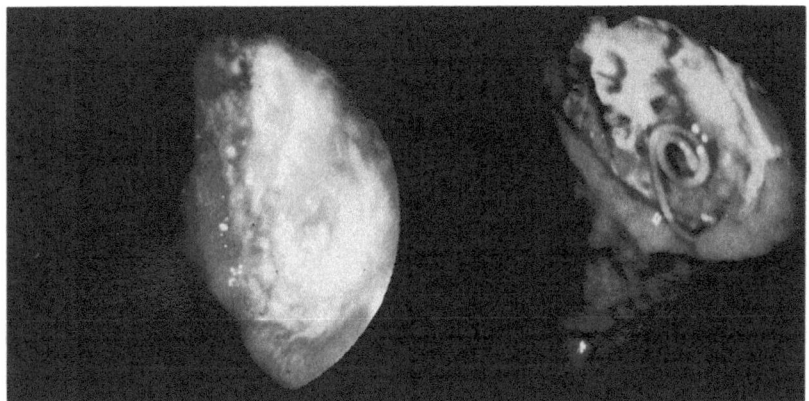

a   b

Fig. 5. a A large ulcer at the posterior wall of the angulus of the stomach detected by endoscopic examination. **b** A larva penetrating the ulcer floor demonstrated by means of the contrast-dye method on endoscopic examination

Case 2

The patient (57 year-old male) suffered from hunger pains from 20 August 1984, but after taking medication no symptoms occurred for over 2 weeks prior to endoscopic examination on 11 September 1984. We found two large ulcers at the angulus of the stomach (Fig. 5a). By means of the contrast-dye method, a larva was discovered penetrating the ulcer foor at the posterior wall of the angulus, but this was not evident before application of the dye solution (Fig. 5b). Resection was performed by endoscopic biopsy forceps and the preparation was histologically identified as *Anisakis simplex* larva.

Discussion

In many cases of acute gastric anisakiasis, X-ray examination reveals widening of the gastric angle and/or swollen mucosal folds, and a larva is usually seen as a radiolucent thin thread [6]. Recently, however, endoscopic examination has been used because a larva can be more easily detected in addtion to being resectable by biopsy forceps. Many cases have been reported where *Anisakis* larvae could be removed by biopsy forceps and thereafter the syptoms quickly disappeared. On the other hand, there are several cases in which patients possess the symptoms suggesting acute gastric anisakiasis but lack evidence of an *Anisakis* larva upon endoscopic examination. In these cases, the contrast-dye method is very useful for demonstrating the presence of the larva. Nishimura et al. [7] reported a case in which gastric anisakiasis was suspected but a larva could not be found on routine endoscopic examination but was discovered easily using the contrast-dye method. Even if a larva is evident in the routine endoscopic examination, we believe the contrast-dye method to be a superior technique because it allows other larvae to be detected.

We have experienced two cases of anisakiasis without acute gastrointestinal symptoms in which the existence of a larva was unexpectedly confirmed by the contrast-dye method on endoscopic examination, suggesting additional value of this method.

As the contrast-dye method is very useful for detecting the *Anisakis* larva, this technique may prove to be the best when examining patients with the endoscope who have complaints connected with gastric anisakiasis.

References

1. Namiki T, Morooka T, Kawauchi H, Ueda N, Sekiya C, Nakagawa K, Furuta T, Ooguro T, Kamada H (1970) Diagnosis of acute gastric anisakiasis. Stomach Intestine 5: 1437–1440 (in Japanese)
2. Tashiro N, Katagiri J, Aikawa K (1983) Studies on endoscopic pictures of gastric anisakiases. Gastroenterol Endosc 25: 1118 (in Japanese)
3. Aoki S (1968) Endoscopic study on gastric ulcer and scar using dye-spreading method. Gastroenterol Endosc 10: 202–217 (in Japanese)
4. Ida K, Hashimoto Y, Takeda S, Murakami K, Kawai K (1975) Endoscopic diagnosis of gastric cancer with dye scattering. Am J Gastroenterol 63: 316–320
5. Hoshihara Y, Yamamoto T, Koyama M, Kawahara H, Kawaguchi Y, Watanabe K (1984) A case of gastric anisakiasis without acute gastrointestinal symptoms, unexpectedly found by contrast dye-method on the endoscopic examination. Prog Digest Endosc 25: 223–225 (in Japanese)
6. Kawauchi H, Namiki T, Morooka T, Nakagawa K, Ooguro T (1973) Gastric anisakiasis presenting acute gastrointestinal symptoms—with special reference to the endoscopic and roentgenographic findings of *Anisakis* larva penetrating into the wall of the human stomach and to its clinical features. Stomach Intestine 8: 31–38 (in Japanese)
7. Nishimura T, Sano R, Komatsu T, Fukuma T, Shinka S, Kojima T, Tabata B (1981) Studies on anisakiasis in south-western district of Hyogo prefecture (II). Jpn J Parasitol 30: 53 (in Japanese)

Serological and Immunological Studies

M. Tsuji

General Remarks

It is well known that in *Anisakis* infections remarkable eosinophilic infiltrations are seen in the tissue surrounding the larvae and that the imbedded area of the worms shows a strong allergic reaction. A reliable diagnosis of anisakiasis depends on recovery of the worms. The morphological examinations, however, are not easy and are often very difficult in chronic cases or where there is a latent clinical symptomatology.

In the past several years, a considerable amount of work on serological studies has been performed for the diagnosis of anisakiasis, such as the complement fixation test, indirect hemagglutination test, Ouchterlony and immunoelectrophoresis, indirect fluorescene test, latex agglutination test, and enzyme-linked immunosorbent assay. The results have indicated that positive serological tests for anisakiasis are closely connected with the survival of worms in the patients, but the tests have not included cross reactivity with other nematode infections [1]. In the studies described in this chapter, an attempt was made to determin practical values for the diagnosis and critera for treatment on the basis of serological tests.

Cross Reactions Between *Anisakis* and Other Nematodes

Antiserum was prepared by immunizing rabbits with *Anisakis* larvae and female adult worms collected from mackerel and dolphins and antigens from six species of nematodes. A reverse combination of antigen and antiserum was used for immunoelectrophoresis. As an antigen, 0.1% saline extract of the worms was used, and 0.9% agarose in veronal buffered saline (pH 8.2) was used as the plate [2].

The results are shown in Tables 1 and 2. The serum of a rabbit immunized with *Anisakis* larvae obtained from mackerel showed 24 bands with *Anisakis* larvae (mackerel) antigen, 16 bands with larvae from a dolphin, and 14 bands with female adults from a dolphin.

In the sera derived from immunization with *Anisakis* larvae (mackerel), 12 bands each were demonstrated of cross reaction with *Ascaris suum* female, *Ascaris suum* male, *Ascaris lumbricoides* female, and *Toxocara canis* female

Table 1. Cross reactions between hyperimmune sera of *Anisakis* and other nematode antigens by immunoelectrophoresis

Antisera	*Anisakis* larvae (mackerel)	*Anisakis* larvae (dolphin)	*Anisakis* female adults	*Ascaris suum* female	*Ascaris suum* male	*Ascaris lumbrico-ides* female	*Ascaris lumbrico-ides* male	*Toxocara canis* female	*Angiostrongylus cantonensis* female	*Angiostrongylus cantonensis* male	*Dirofilaria immitis*
Anisakis larvae (mackerel)	24	16	14	12	12	12	11	12	9	8	9
Anisakis larvae (dolphin)	16	24	15	12	11	12	11	12	8	8	8
Anisakis female adults (dolphin)	14	15	20	9	8	8	8	15	8	8	9

Table 2. Cross reactions between *Anisakis* antigens and hyperimmune sera of other nematodes by immunoelectrophoresis

Antigens	*Anisakis* larvae (mackerel)	*Anisakis* larvae (dolphin)	*Anisakis* female adults	*Ascaris suum* female	*Ascaris suum* male	*Ascaris lumbrico-ides* female	*Ascaris lumbrico-ides* male	*Toxocara canis* female	*Angiostrongylus cantonensis* female	*Angiostrongylus cantonensis* male	*Dirofilaria immitis*
Anisakis larvae (mackerel)	24	16	14	12	11	11	11	12	9	7	5
Anisakis larvae (dolphin)	16	24	15	12	11	11	11	12	9	8	6
Anisakis female adults (dolphin)	14	15	20	7	7	8	7	12	9	8	6

antigens, 11 bands with *Ascaris lumbricoides* male, nine bands each with *Angio-strongylus cantonensis* female and *Dirofilaria immitis*, and eight bands with *Angiostrongylus cantonensis* male antigen.

The reverse reactions, i.e., the reactions between *Anisakis* larvae (mackerel) antigen and the rabbit sera immunized with other nematodes, virtually paralleled those shown in Tables 1 and 2. Namely, *Anisakis* larvae (mackerel) antigen showed 12 bands each with the immunized rabbit sera of *Ascaris suum* female and *Toxocara canis* female, 11 bands each with the antisera of *Ascaris suum* male, *Ascaris lumbricoides* female and male, nine bands with *Angiostrongylus cantonensis* female, seven bands with *Angiostrongylus cantonensis* male, and five bands with *Dirofilaria immitis* antisera.

It can be said from the results that many common bands of nematodes exist, and the strongest reactions were observed between the antigen and its homologous antisera.

Immunoelectrophoregrams of *Anisakis* Antigen and Its Hyperimmune Sera

Immunoelectrophoregrams of *Anisakis* larvae collected from mackerel and dolphins and *Anisakis* female adults from dolphins are shown in Fig.1.

Interpretation of such patterns is very difficult and can only be resolved by repeating the experiment with the absorption technique. Absorption should be done with care. One milliliter of the hyperimmune rabbit serum of *Anisakis*

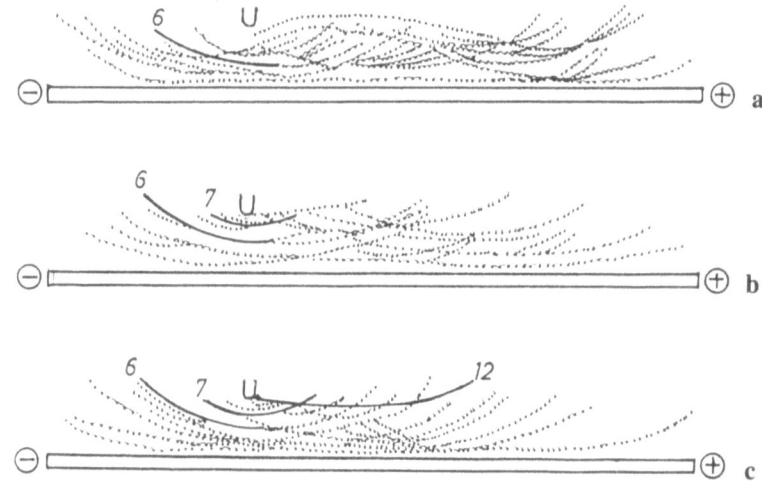

Fig. 1a–c. Antigenic structure and specific bands of genus *Anisakis*. **a** *Anisakis* larvae (from mackerel) antigen and anti-*Anisakis* larvae (from mackerel) serum. **b** *Anisakis* larvae (from dolphin) antigen and anti-*Anisakis* larvae (from dolphin) serum. **c** *Anisakis* adult female antigen and anti-*Anisakis* adult female serum. Band *6* specific for genus *Anisakis*, band *7* specific for *Anisakis* from dolphin, band *12* specific for *Anisakis* adult. *Dotted lines* indicate common bands with other genus antigens

Table 3. Results of diagnosis for helminthic diseases by serological tests

Chief complaint or clinical symptoms	No. examinations	No. positive	
Eosinophilia	72	33	*Anis.* 3, *T. can* 20, *T. cat* 5, *F. hep* 2, *U. col* 3
Gastrointestinal complaint	142	60	*Anis.* 39, *S. ster* 1, *E. panc* 1, *M. yoko* 2, *D. lat* 1, *T. sag* 1, *U. col* 12, Crohn 2, *P. nod* 1
Liver complaint	58	16	*T. can* 5, *C. sin* 5, *S. jap* 2, *E. mul* 2, *U. col* 1, *P. nod* 1
Nervous complaint	16	4	*T.can* 2, *A. canto* 2
Lung complaint	96	31	*P. west* 23, *P. miya* 3, *P. nod* 5
Cutaneous or muscle symptom	46	9	*G. spin* 2, *S. erin* 6, *U. col* 1
Chyluria	8	0	
Others	23	4	*E. mul* 2, *P. nod* 2
Total	461	157	

Anis. Anisakis, *T. can* Toxocara canis, *T. cat* Toxocara cati, *A. cant* Angiostrongylus cantonensis, *S. ster* Strongylus stercolaris, *G. spin* Gnathostoma spinigerum, *F. hep* Fasciola hepatica, *C. sin* Clonorchis sinensis, *E. panc* Eurytrema pancreaticum, *P. west* Paragonimus westermani, *P. miya* Paragonimus miyazakii, *S. jap* Schistosoma japonicum, *M. yoko* Metagonimus yokogawai, *D. lat* Diphyllobothrium latum, *S. erin* Spirometra erinacei, *T. sag* Taenia saginata, *E. mul* Echinococcus multiloculars, *U. col* Ulcerative colitis, *Crohn* Crohn's disease, *P. nod* Periarteritis nodosa

larvae was absorbed with 20 mg of another nematode antigen. After stirring, the antiserum-antigen mixture was incubated for 3 h at 37°C, then stored and refrigerated for 12–24 h. The dotted lines in Fig. 1 disappeared upon absorption, and bands 6, 7, and 12 were recognized as the residual reaction of anti-*Anisakis* serum after absorption. It can be said from these diagrams that band 6 is the common precipitation of the genus *Anisakis* and band 12 is the specific precipitation for *Anisakis* adults. These specific bands were recognized in the sera of 82% of anisakiasis patients but were never checked in the cases of other nematode infections.

Clinical Trials of Serological Tests

As a routine examination in our laboratory, 461 patients who had various complaints were tested by serological tests in 1984. Of the 461 cases, 157 were shown to be positive for a helminthic antigen, as shown in Table 3.

Three cases had a specific band of *Anisakis* upon immunoelectrophoresis (IEP) in the group of eosinophilia, and one of them was pathologically proved to be an *Anisakis* larva after being removed from the stomach by operation. Another 39 patients who had a gastrointestinal complaint such as abdominal

Table 4. Numbers of positive cases for serological tests by helminthic antigens

	Positive	Morph.	Serol. test neg.
Nematodes			
Anisakis larvae	42	25	7
T. canis	27		
T. cati	5		
S. stercoralis	1	1	
A. cantonensis	2		
G. spinigerum	2		
Trematodes			
F. hepatica	2	1	
C. sinensis	5	1	1
E. pancreaticum	1	1	
P. westermani	23	1	
P. miyazakii	3		
S. japonicum	2	2	7
M. yokogawai	2	2	1
Cestodes			
D. latum	1	1	
S. erinacei	6	1	
T. saginata	1	1	2
E. multilocularis	4		
Other diseases			
Ulcerative colitis	17		
Crohn's disease	2		
Periarteritis nodosa	9		

Morph. positive for morphological examinations, *Serol. test neg.* positive for morphology but negative for serological tests

pain or granuloma formation were shown to be positive in the complement fixation test (CFT), indirect fluorescent antibody test (IFA), and/or Ouchterlony (DDT) and IEP.

In 12 cases, the progress was observed without giving any treatment. Three to seven months later, their antibodies became negative, and all eosinophilia, complaints, and symptoms disappeared. These cases should be suspected as being anisakiasis.

Seropositives were detected in 25 of 42 cases of *Anisakis* larvae by endoscopic examination, but seven cases were negative in serotests even though *Anisakis* larvae were found, as shown in Table 4. But all of these cases became positive after one month. This occurrence of this phenomenon was seen to depend on the time of bleeding.

Serological Results of Primary Infection Cases

In the cases of primary infection, the first positive reactions were recognized 10–25 days after infection in CFT, 10–20 days in indirect hemagglutination test (IHA), 10–35 days in DDT and IEP, 10–30 days in IFA, and 10–20 days in

Table 5. Antibody production in the sera of anisakiasis patients as detected in various tests

	Positive rate (%)	First positive (days after infection)	Became negative (months after infection)
Complement fixation test	85	10–25	1–12
Hemagglutination test	85	10–20	1–15
Immunoelectrophoresis	95	10–35	2–18
Indirect immunofluorescence test (IgG)	95	10–30	2–15
Enzyme-linked immunosorbent assay	95	10–20	1–12

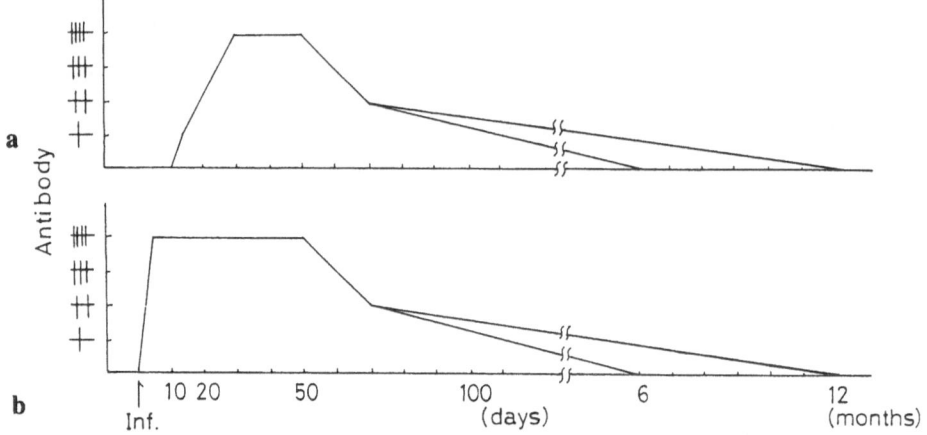

Fig. 2a, b. Changes of antibody titers in I.E.P. in cases of anisakiasis. **a** Primary infection, **b** reinfection

enzyme-linked immunosorbent assay (ELISA), as shown in Table 5 and Fig. 2. In follow-up examinations, the antibody titers of these tests increased, and the maximum titers were recognized at 3–10 weeks after infection at the time when the granuloma had developed; these titers then showed a tendency to decrease slowly and finally became negative after 1–18 months. CFT and ELISA results became negative faster than the other techniques 1–12 months after infection; results in IHA became negative after 1–15 months, IFA after 2–15 months, and DDT and IEP after 2–18 months.

Serological Results of Reinfection Cases

In the cases of reinfection, the first positive reactions were recognized 6–24 h after infection, as shown in Fig. 2. Even in the cases where the *Anisakis* larvae was removed endoscopically, the antibodies increased immediately and showed maximum titers. It is possible that the excretions of the invading *Anisakis* larvae boost the effects of the antibody. Changes in the antibody titers in the follow-up examination were the same as in the primary infection cases.

Positive Rate of Each Test

The positive rate in serological tests was 85%–95% in anisakiasis patients. In CFT and IHA, the positive rate was about 85%, in DDT about 90%, in IEP, IFA, and ELISA about 95%. However, in the cases of primary infection, the antibody titers were not checked in spite of the worms being detected as previously described. These cases should undergo follow-up examination. With regard to the problem of cross reactivity, the strongest reactions were observed between the antigen and its homologous antisera in all tests. The antigens of related species should be diagnosed for differentiation. The detection of a specific band of *Anisakis* by IEP is also very useful in the diagnosis of anisakiasis.

In conclusion, the serological diagnosis for anisakiasis should be conducted simultaneously with several tests, and the positive serological tests for anisakiasis are closely connected with survival of the worms in the patients. Serological tests are very useful parameters for the diagnosis, assessment, and cure of anisakiasis.

References

1. Desowitz RS (1986) Human and experimental anisakiasis in the United States. Hokkaido Igaku Zasshi 61(3): 358–371
2. Tsuji M (1975) Comparative studies on the antigenic structure of several helminths by immunoelectrophoresis. Jpn J Parasitol 24(4): 227–236 (in Japanese)

Latex Agglutination Test for Immunodiagnosis of Gastric Anisakiasis

N. AKAO and H. YOSHIMURA

Introduction

Recent advances in gastroendoscopic examination have led to the easy detection and removal of *Anisakis* larvae. This technique is widely used to diagnose gastric anisakiasis in Japan. In some patients with severe abdominal pain, however, we have often experienced that the parasite was not detected with this technique. This may be because the parasite has already escaped from the stomach to the intestine or penetrated the gastric mucosal layer.

Since the *Anisakis* larva elicits a host immune response, many investigators have attempted to develop more sensitive and specific immunodiagnostic techniques [1–5]. Over the past decade, we have been using a latex agglutination test (LA) in experimentally infected animals and human cases [6–7]. The present chapter covers our current results and presents a discussion of the advantages and disadvantages of this test for clinical trials.

Subjects of Investigation

Patients

From February 1975 to March 1986, antibody titers of 1249 patients sera with characteristic clinical symptoms were assayed by LA. Of them, 553 were confirmed as being gastric anisakiasis. Of the 553 patients, 150 (93 males, 54 females, and three unknown) were proven cases with one or more larvae of *Anisakis simplex* (L3) and 14 (five males and nine females) had one larva of *Pseudoterranova decipiens*. Almost all the worms were removed or detected by gastroendoscopic examination. The remaining 388 cases were not proven but suspected as gastric anisakiasis based on their clinical symptoms.

Control

Control sera were obtained from healthy adults aged 18–65 years old. A total of 320 sera were examined.

Antigen and Procedure of LA

Antigen

Somatic antigen of *Anisakis simplex* larvae was prepared by the modified procedure of Suzuki et al. (1969 [8]). Briefly, the worms were taken from mackerel and incubated in artificial gastric juice (0.5% 1:1000 pepsin, 0.7% hydrochloric acid) for 1 h at 37°C. They were then extensively washed three times in distilled water and phosphate buffered saline (PBS; pH 7.2). After removal of excessive PBS on paper filter, the worms were frozen at −80°C and dried by vaccum-drying equipment (Yamato Freeze-dryer, Model DC-35, Yamato Scientific Co., Ltd., Tokyo, Japan). The worms were cut into small pieces and mashed with a mortar and pestle. Then, the frozen powder was sonicated in ten volumes of PBS using an ultrasound disrupter (Tomy Seiko Co., Ltd., Tokyo, Japan) at 160 W for 5 min on ice. The product was centrifuged for 1 h at $10\,000 \times g$. The supernatant was collected and sterilized by membrane filtration through a 0.22-μm-pore membrane (Nihon Millipore Kogyo Co., Ltd., Yonezawa, Japan). Finally, the sterilized supernatant was dialyzed against distilled water and centrifuged. This product was lyophilized and designated as *Anisakis* antigen. To examine the cross reactivity, the following antigens were also prepared by the procedures in addition to *Anisakis* antigen—*Ascaris suum* adult female, *Toxocara canis* adult female, and *Dirofilaria immitis* adult female.

Preparation of Latex Particles and Procedure of LA

The antigens were reconstituted in 0.2 M ammonium chloride ammonium buffer solution (pH 8.0) to achieve a protein concentration of 0.37 mg/ml. The protein content of the antigens was determined by the method of Lowry et al. [9]. One volume of the 0.5% emulsion-containing polystyrene latex particles (0.9 μm in diameter, Takeda Pharm. Co., Ltd., Tokyo, Japan) was suspended in the same buffer, and the particles were sensitized with two volumes of each antigen solution. The time required for antigen sensitization was 60 min at 37°C. Using the same buffer solution, the sensitized latex antigens were washed and centrifuged twice to remove the excess antigen. The sensitized latex antigens were resuspended to a concentration of 0.1% in addition to the same buffer solution supplemented with 0.5% weight/volume bovine serum albumin. Thus, the final latex antigens were used for immunodiagnosis of anisakiasis. (These reagents were kindly supplied by Dr. Tubota, Research Laboratory, Eiken Chemical Co., Ltd., Tokyo, Japan.)

LA was performed according to the procedure of Tubota and Ozawa [10]. A V-shaped microtiter plate was used in this study, except where otherwise stated.

Seropositivity in Healthy Subjects and Patients

Frequency distribution of the LA titer in controls and the two patient groups is shown in Fig. 1. The patient groups showed bimodal antibody curves, whereas these were unimodal in controls. Distribution of the LA titer in controls over-

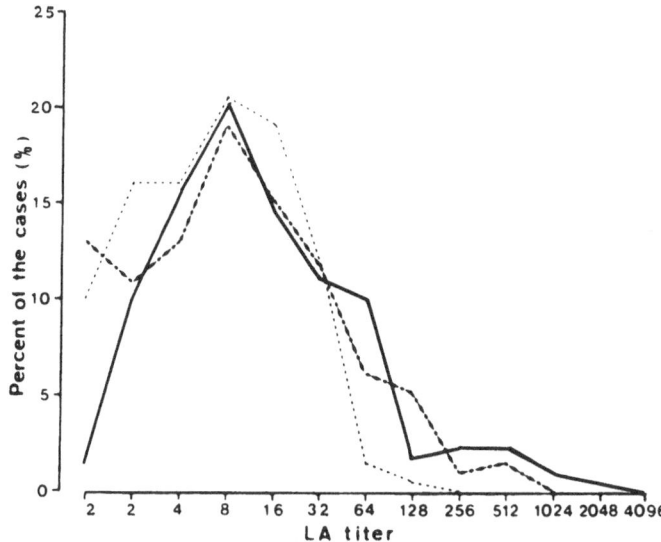

Fig. 1. Frequency distribution of the titers in the latex agglutination test in proven cases (——), suspected cases (·······), and controls (------)

lapped with that of the LA titer in the patient groups, suggesting the existence of an occult infection or a presensitized state in the control group. When an LA titer of 1:128 or more was considered positive, 1.3% of the control sera were classed as false positive. In both patient groups, however, there was an increase of positivity at the high titers; conversely, no sera were found with an LA titer of more than 1:1024 among the controls. However, the reciprocal of the mean $\log_2$ titers against *Anisakis* antigen in proven cases, suspected cases, and controls were 4.13 ± 2.61, 3.40 ± 2.38, and 2.79 ± 1.74, respectively, with no significant differences among the three groups. Cross reactivity to three helminthic antigens is shown in Table 1. The sera of the patient groups cross-reacted with all these antigens.

In a previous study, we demonstrated that the antibody levels of proven cases in gastric anisakiasis were significantly higher than in controls [11]. The discrepancy between these results may be due to the time lag in the taking of blood after onset. In the early 1970s, gastroendoscopic examination was not so common, and many cases may have been frequently misdiagnosed. Therefore, antibody levels in the sera were higher at the time they were brought to our laboratory. At present, most cases are diagnosed fairly well endoscopically. Sera are taken immediately after the onset; accordingly, it would seem that the antibody to *Anisakis* antigen is not sufficiently produced at such a time.

Suzuki et al. [3] studied two groups of people in a small town in Hokkaido by means of an indirect hemagglutination test (IHA). In one group of 21 proven cases of gastric anisakiasis, the seropositivity rate was 95.2%; by contrast, a seropositivity rate of 30.8% was found in 500 healthy persons. Therefore, they concluded that IHA was not useful in the serodiagnosis of gastric anisakiasis. From our results, we would agree with their conclusions, but we noted that there were some patients with a high anti-*Anisakis* antibody level of not less than 1:1024 who had gastric anisakiasis.

Table 1. Comparisons of titers of latex agglutination to four different nematode antigens in proven cases, clinically suspected cases, and normal controls

	Latex agglutination titer against			
	Anisakis	*Ascaris*	*Toxocara*	*Dirofilaria*
Proven cases	4.13 ± 2.60(164)	2.43 ± 1.06 (98)	2.95 ± 1.38(106)	2.91 ± 1.33 (35)
Suspected cases	3.40 ± 2.38(388)	2.58 ± 1.20(164)	3.20 ± 1.51(171)	2.86 ± 1.34 (58)
Controls	2.79 ± 1.74(320)	2.05 ± 1.17(320)	2.13 ± 1.34(320)	1.78 ± 1.20(320)

Parentheses indicate number of sera examined
Figures are given as means $\log_2$ titer $\pm$ SD

Follow-up Study of LA in Gastric Anisakiasis

From the above combined results, it can be seen that only one examination of sera in patients was not reliable because of the presence of false-negative factors in the two patient groups and false-positive results in the controls. Moreover, there are some cases of acute gastric anisakiasis which have low antibody titers even though the parasite is found. Thus, we evaluated the follow-up study using paired sera taken after an interval of time (Table 2). In proven cases, a total of 28 paired sera were examined; six of them were collected within 6 days and 22 more than 6 days after the first test. Significant elevation of the antibody titer was observed in more than half of the sera in the latter group. However, antibody levels in seven of these cases were unchanged. The penetrating worms in these cases had already been removed by gastroendoscopy within 2 days of onset. Therefore, it may be that the antibody titer detected by LA was not be elevated in these seven cases. This tendency was also observed in clinically suspected cases: Of 69 paired sera, the number of cases showing a significant increase in antibody level was 26 in sera taken 6 days after the first test and two in sera taken within 6 days. It was confirmed that the paired sera examination was effective. Ruitenberg [5] noted that the patient sera should be examined at least twice in the course of the disease, with an interval of 3 or 4 weeks after the first examination.

These results coincided with those in an animal model. We demonstrated antibody response in rabbits experimentally infected with *Anisakis* larvae using LA and the double-gel diffusion test [7]. In primary infection, LA antibody was detected 1 week after infection; a significant elevation of antibody titer was then seen 3 days after secondary infection.

Conclusion

Since immunogloblin classes reflected on LA are IgG and IgM, a specific IgA or IgE antibody has been neglected. Recently, Desowitz et al. [12] demonstrated that specific IgE antibody against *Anisakis* antigen was elevated in anisakiasis patients using a radioallergosorbent test. We [7] previously reported that the

Table 2. Follow-up study of titers to *Anisakis* antigen in the latex agglutination test with proven and suspected cases

Change in antibody levels between 1st and 2nd exam.	Within 6 days[a]				More than 6 days[a]			
	Proven cases	Suspected cases	Total	Percent	Proven cases	Suspected cases	Total	Percent
Fourfold or more	1	2	3	21.4	8	26	34	41.0
Twofold	1	3	4	28.6	6	5	11	18.2
Unchanged	4	3	7	50.0	7	22	29	34.9
Half or less	0	0	0	0.0	1	8	9	10.8

[a] The period is that from the first examination to the second

specific IgA antibody level was increased in proven cases of anisakiasis. Additional work is required to clarify the significance of these findings.

The procedure in LA is simpler than in other immunodiagnostic tests, and the latex reagent is more stable than the tannic acid-treated sheep erythrocytes in IHA. Though the *Anisakis* antigen used in this study was not always specific, the antigen showed extensive cross reactivity against other helminth antigens [2, 5–7, 11, 13, 14]. To solve this problem, further study of purification of the antigen is needed. Suzuki et al. [8] demonstrated that the hemoglobin fraction of *Anisakis* larval extracts was a specific antigen, and the fraction did not show cross reactivity with other nematodes.

In spite of the existence of cross reactivity, LA appears to be suitable for clinical immunodiagnosis of human gastric anisakiasis.

References

1. Kobayashi A, Kumada M, Ishizaki T, Katuro T, Koito K (1968) Skin tests with somatic and ES (excretions and secretions) antigens from *Anisakis* larvae: II. The difference of antigenicity between the two antigens. Jpn J Parasitol 17: 414–418 (in Japanese)
2. Suzuki T, Shiraki T, Sekino T, Otsuru M, Ishikura H (1970) Studies on the immunological diagnosis of anisakiasis: III. Intradermal test with purified antigen. Jpn J Parasitol 19: 1–9 (in Japanese)
3. Suzuki T, Ishida K, Ishigooka K, Doi K, Otsuru M, Sato R, Asaishi K, Nishino C (1975) Studies on the immunological diagnosis of anisakiasis: V. Intradermal and indirect hemagglutination tests, and histopathological examination of biopsied mucous membranes on gastric anisakiasis. Jpn J Parasitol 24: 184–191 (in Japanese)
4. Suzuki T, Ishida K, Asaishi K, Nishino C (1976) Studies on the immunodiagnosis of anisakiasis: VI. Analysis of criteria on intradermal and indirect hemagglutination tests by means of radioimmunoassay. Jpn J Parasitol 25: 17–23 (in Japanese)
5. Ruitenberg EJ (1970) Anisakiasis. Pathogenesis, Serodiagnosis and prevention (Monograph). Rijksuniversiteit, Utrecht, pp 55–66
6. Yoshimura H, Kondo K, Ohnishi Y, Akao N, Tubota N (1978) Summary of the cases of *Anisakis* infections during past three years, with special reference to clinicopathology and immunodiagnoses. Nippon Iji Sinpo 2837: 29–32 (in Japanese)
7. Yoshimura H, Kondo K, Ohnishi Y, Akao N (1983) Studies on immunodiagnosis of anisakiasis. Report for Scientific Research Grant from Ministry of Education of

Japan, pp 13–28 (in Japanese)
8. Suzuki T, Shirakawa T, Otsuru M (1969) Studies on the immunodiagnoisis of anisa-kiasis: II. Isolation and purification of *Anisakis* antigen. Jpn J Parasitol 18: 232–240 (in Japanese)
9. Lowry OH, Rosebrough NJ, Farr AL, Randall RJ (1951) Protein measurement with Folin phenol reagent. J Biol Chem 193: 265–275
10. Tubota N, Ozawa H (1977) Studies on latex agglutination test for toxoplasmosis: I. Preparative conditions and stability of the reagent. Jpn J Parasitol 26: 276–285 (in Japanese)
11. Yoshimura H, Akao N, Kondo K, Ohnishi Y, Funaoka H, Yamane K (1980) Two cases of extragastrointestinal anisakiasis and evaluation of immunodiagnosis. Jpn J Clin Pathol 28: 708–712 (in Japanese)
12. Desowitz RS, Raybourne RB, Ishikura H, Kliks MM (1985) The radioallergosorbent test (RAST) for the serological diagnosis of human anisakiasis. Trans Roy Soc Trop Med Hyg 79: 256–259
13. Oshima T (1972) *Anisakis* and anisakiasis in Japan and adjacent area. In: Morishitak, Komiya Y, Matsubayashi H (eds) Progress of Medical Parasitology in Japan, vol. 4, Meguro Parasitological Museum, Tokyo, pp 301–393
14. Smith JW, Wootten R (1978) *Anisakis* and Anisakiasis. In: Lumsden WHR (ed) Advances in Parasitology, vol. 16. Academic, London. pp 93–163

Monoclonal Antibody, Intradermal Reaction, and Sarles' Phenomenon

S. Takahashi, H. Ishikura, and H. Hayasaka

Introduction

There have been a considerable number of reports in which the antigens of *Anisakis simplex* larvae were analyzed by using xenogenic serum. However, it is still difficult to detect specific antigens of the worm because of the high degree of cross reactivities of the antiserum with other nematodes such as *Pseudoterranova decipiens* larva. The recent success with monoclonal antibodies has led to the production of very specific antibodies in many areas of parasitology. In the present study, we developed hybridomas to obtain monoclonal antibodies for the purpose of detecting the specific antigens present in *Anisakis* larvae. In this attempt, it has become possible to detect specific epitopes of larvae, distinguishing them from other nematodes, and to analyze the corresponding antigens biochemically. It is obviously important to detect specific antigens of *Anisakis* larvae in the study of the taxonomic features of anisakid species and the pathological aspects ofanisakiasis. This approach may also lead to improvement in the specificity of the enzyme-linked immunosorbent assay (ELISA) as a serodiagnostic test for anisakiasis.

Hybridoma Production

Antigen Preparation and Immunization of Mice

Anisakis larvae were taken from the viscera of Alaska pollack in the Sea of Japan around Hokkaido. They were homogenized in phosphate buffered saline (PBS), centrifuged at 3000 rpm twice for 10 min, and the supernatants were collected. The supernatants were prepared for both the immunization of mice and solid-phase antigens in ELISA for screening of the hybridoma cell line. The supernatents were also prepared for biochemical analysis of specific antigens using monoclonal antibodies.

Balb/c mice were immunized intraperitoneally with 200 μg of prepared antigens at weekly intervals for 5 weeks. The mouse serum as tested for positive antibody generation against the worm on frozen sections by the indirect immunofluorescence (IF) technique.

Hybridoma Procedure

The hybridization experiment was carried out as described by Kohler and Milstein [1]. The immunized spleen was minced and suspended in plain RPMI-1640 medium and washed twice. Approximately 10^8 spleen cells were mixed with 2×10^7 NS-1 mouse myeloma cells, and the mixture was centrifuged at 800 rpm for 10 min. The cell pellet was resuspended by gently tapping and was left in 0.2 ml polyethylene glycol for 2 min; it was then diluted in drips of 8 ml plain RPMI-1640 medium. The cells were centrifuged again and resuspended in a solution of complete medium containing hypoxanthine (1×10^{-4} mol/l), aminopterine (4×10^{-7} mol/l), thymidine (1.6×10^5 mol/l), and 10% heat-inactivated fetal bovine serum. After incubating for several hours, the cells were seeded into 24-well plates with spleen cells from normal mice as feeder cells. The hybridomas growing in the wells were first checked on the 7th day of cultivation. The production of antibodies directed against *Anisakis* larvae was assessed with ELISA and IF tests. ELISA was performed using a microELISA plate (Immulon2, Dynatech Laboratories Inc.). The prepared antigen of *Anisakis* larvae and *Ascaris suum* was applied to the plates, and the hybridomas reactive only to *Anisakis* larvae were selected. These were immediately cloned by limiting dilution.

Specificity and Localization of Antigens Defined by Monoclonal Antibodies

Seven of 157 hybridomas were selected for cloning. They were all found to produce antibodies against *Anisakis* larvae but not against *Ascaris suum* in ELISA (Fig. 1). Furthermore, they did not show any cross reactivity with *Echinococcus multilocularis. Pseudoterranova decipiens*, *Trichinella spiralis. Dirofilaria immitis. Toxocara cati.* and *Ascaris suum* in IF tests. The patterns of reactivity with monoclonal antibodies on frozen sections of *Anisakis* larvae are shown in (Fig. 2) and summarized in Table 1. Among these monoclonal antibodies, An2, An6, and An7 are supposed to be related to excretory-secretory (E-S) antigens because of their reactivity with Renette cells and the intestine. Thereafter, An2 and An6 were investigated as to their reactivity with E-S antigens using ELISA. As shown in Fig. 3, An2 and An6 reacted to E-S antigens; An2 especially was highly reactive to the early phase of the antigens. Although they are not fully understood as yet, E-S antigens are thought to be released during sloughing. However, our results showed that some E-S antigens at least are secreted actively from live *Anisakis* larvae.

Molecular Analysis of Antigens

The crude antigen solution was fractionated by gel filtration on a Sephadex G200 column, and reactivity of the monoclonal antibodies against each fraction was screened by ELISA (Fig. 4). Polyacrylamide gel electrophoresis of the antigen in the presence of sodium dodecyl sulfate (SDS-PAGE) and Western blotting of

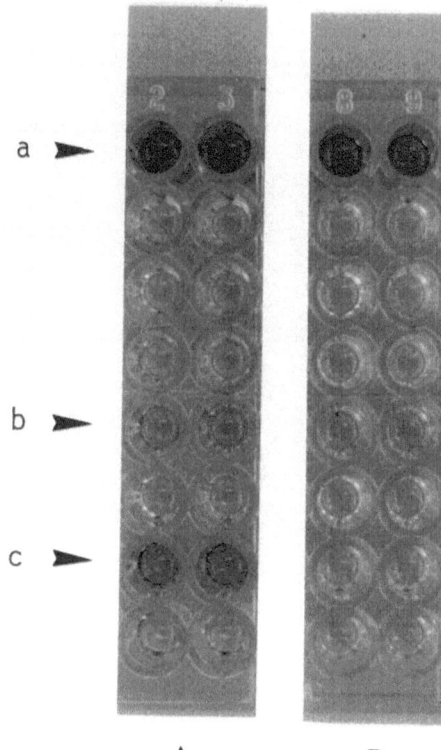

a ➤

b ➤

c ➤

A   B

Fig. 1A, B. ELISA on screening of monoclonal antibodies. Immunized serum showed high reactivities both to **A** *Anisakis* larvae and **B** *Ascaris suum* (*a*). Some of the hybridomas showed cross reactivities against both antigens (*b*). One of the hybridomas showed specific reactivity only to *Anisakis* larvae. This hydridoma was subsequently cloned and designated An2 (*c*)

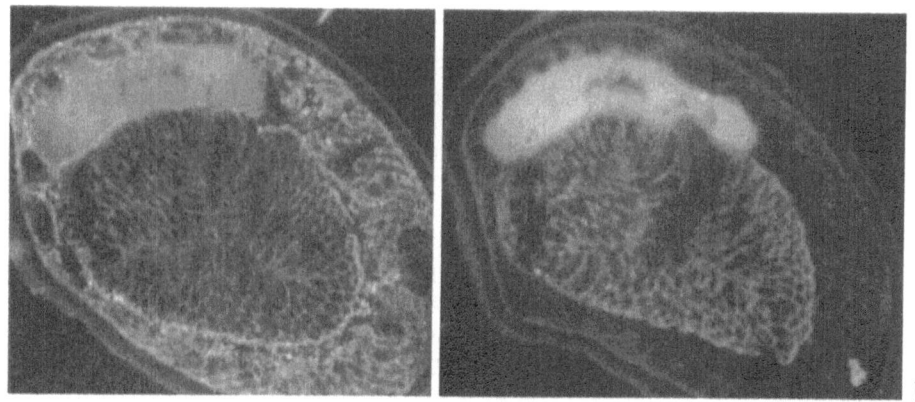

a   b

Fig. 2a, b. Immunofluoroscent staining on frozen sections of *Anisakis* larvae using monoclonal antibodies. **a** An4 showed reactivities to muscle, the Renette cells, and pseudocoel weakly. **b** An7 was reactive to the Renette cells and intestine

Table 1. The patterns of reactivities with monoclonal antibodies on frozen sections of *Anisakis* larvae

Monoclonal antibody	Muscle	Pseudocoel	Renette cells	Intestine	
				Membrane	Cytoplasm
An-1	+	−	+	−	−
An-2	+	±	+	+	−
An-3	+	±	±	−	−
An-4	+	+	+	−	−
An-5	+	±	−	−	−
An-6	+	−	±	−	+
An-7	−	−	+	+	−

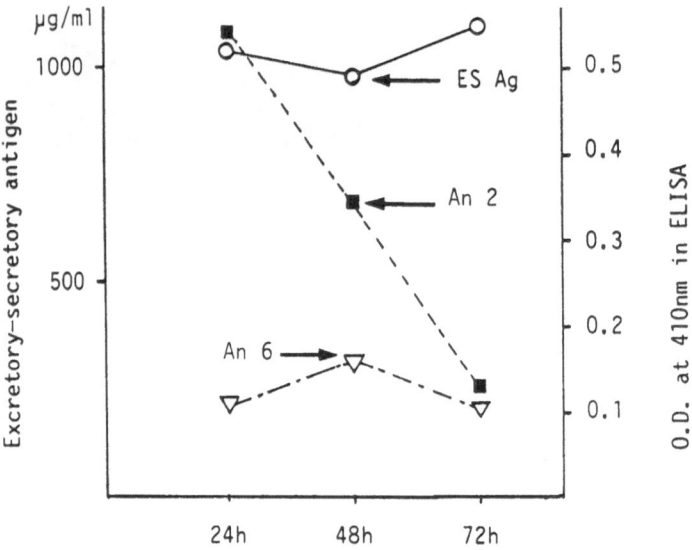

Fig. 3. ELISA against excretory-secretory antigens using monoclonal antibodies. Twenty-five *Anisakis* larvae were incubated in PBS at 37°C and the supernatants were collected. The protein content was measured by Lowry's method. An2 and An6 were reactive against excretory-secretory antigens

the antigen with monoclonal antibodies were also performed. The antigen solution was boiled for 3 min with a sample buffer containing 3% SDS and 5% 2 mercaptoethanol, and electrophoresis of the mixture was done with a 10% polyacrylamide gel. After electrophoresis, the antigen was electrically transferred to Zeta probe membranes (BIO-RAD) and reacted with the monoclonal antibodies. Biotinylated goat antimouse immunoglobulin, peroxidase conjugated avidin, and dianisidine were added. Finally, a dye to detect the bands of corresponding antigens was employed (Fig. 5). The results of these experiments are summarized in Table 2.

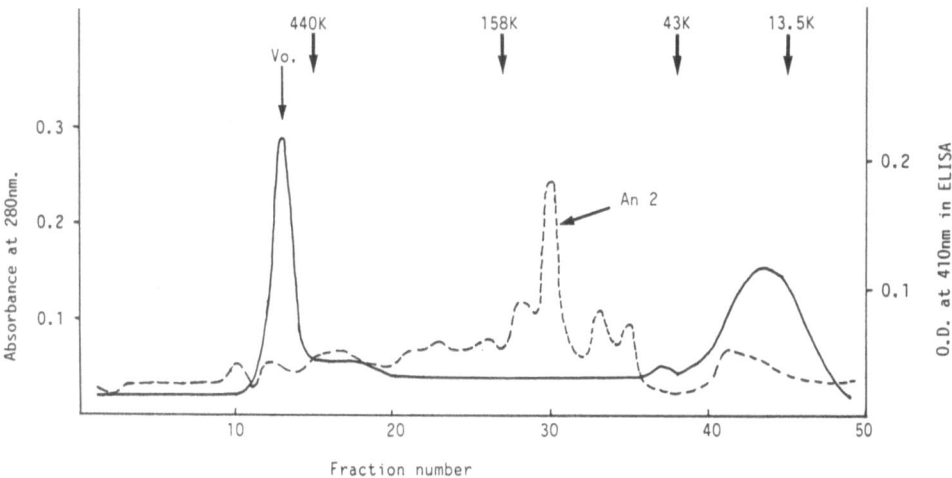

Fig. 4. Antigen solution of *Anisakis* larvae was fractionated by gel filtration, and the reactivities of An2 against each fraction were examined using ELISA. An2 showed reactivity to the protein of about 90 kilodaltons

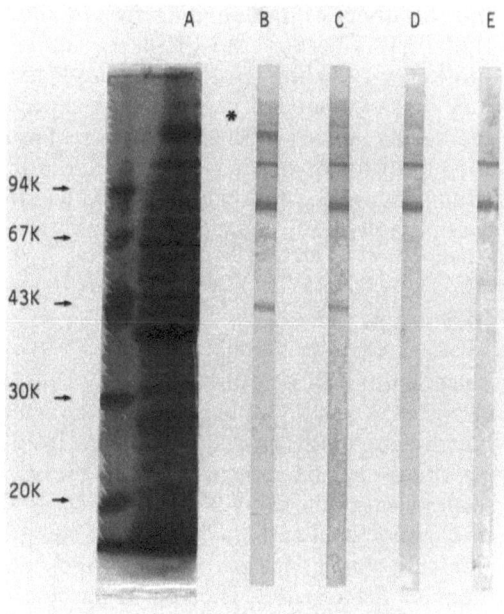

Fig. 5. SDS-PAGE and Western blotting showed that An4 was reactive to the protein of 130 kilodaltons. Lane *A* electrophoresis gel was stained with Coomassie brilliant blue, showing numerous protein bands of the antigen of *Anisakis* larvae; lane *B* An4 detected the protein of 130 kilodaltons (*asterisk*); lane *C* control monoclonal antibody of same subclass; lanes *D* and *E* nonspecific binding of biotinylated antimouse immunoglobulin and peroxidase conjugated avidin, respectively

Table 2. Molecular weight of corresponding antigens reactive against monoclonal antibodies

Monoclonal antibody	Molecular weight of antigen (kilodaltons)
An 1	34 (WB)
An 2	40, 42 (WB)
	90 (GF)
An 3	n.d.
An 4	130 (WB)
An 5	n.d.
An 6	68 (GF)
An 7	n.d.

WB Western blotting, *GF* gel filtration, *n.d.* not determined

Serodiagnositic Applications of Monoclonal Antibodies

A number of techniques such as indirect hemagglutinin tests, immunoprecipitation tests, and radioallergosorbent tests for the immunodiagnosis of anisakiasis have been attempted. However, as of yet, no reliable method for the specificity and sensitivity of immunodiagnosis in anisakiasis has been established. We applied ELISA because of its high sensitivity and potential availability for diverse applications. At first, ELISA with crude antigens of *Anisakis* larvae proved to be very sensitive but not as specific as expected when using polyclonal antiserum against the larvae [2]. The application of monoclonal antibody to ELISA showed an improvement in specificity in addition to preserving the sensitivity. This attempt suggested that the monoclonal antibodies we developed were potentially applicable in serodiagnosis (Fig. 6).

Discussion

Since anisakiasis is a disease clearly caused by *Anisakis* larvae, it is of crucial importance to study the antigenic characteristics of the larvae in understanding the disease mechanism. There have been several important investigations in which the specific antigens of *Anisakis* larvae were studied. However, the antiserum used in these studies showed cross reactivity with other anisakid species. The monoclonal antibody technique has now made it possible to detect the specific antigens of each parasite and to determine their relevance in the development of the disease. The recent success in producing monoclonal antibodies against parasites has been reported for such parasites as *Eimeria tenella* [3], *Leishmania tropica* [4], *Trypanosoma conglense* [5], and *Trichnella spiralis* [6]. Epstein [7] developed a hybridoma that reacted with the stage-specific antigens of malaria. In these studies, monoclonal antibodies contribute in elucidating the mechanism of ontogeny, infectivity, and pathogenesis of the parasites.

In the present study, we extablished seven hybridoma clones that produced monoclonal antibodies which reacted specifically to *Anisakis* larvae. These monoclonals showed different binding patterns on frozen sections of *Anisakis*

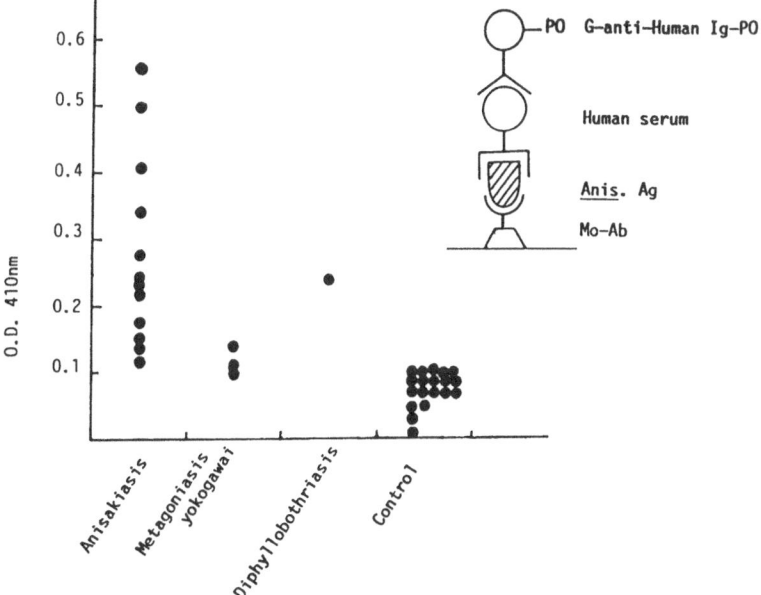

Fig. 6. The results of ELISA using monoclonal antibody (*Mo-Ab*), An2, as shown in the *scheme*. All specimens of the sera were diluted ten times with PBS. There were marked nonspecific reactions using crude antigens of *Anisakis* larvae; however, the reactions of the control sera were minimized by using monoclonal antibody

larvae and did not react with any tissue counterparts or remaining organelles of other species of worms examined. There have been several investigations related to the antigen analysis of *Anisakis* larvae. Agatsuma [8] showed that types I and II of *Anisakis* larvae could be distinguished by enzyme electrophoresis and concluded that this method provides one of the most useful tools other than morphology for identification of the two types of larva. We have not yet examined the reactivity of monoclonal antibodies against *Anisakis physeteris* larvae, but we are convinced that monoclonal antibodies can distinguish between the two types of *Anisakis* larvae using immunostaining.

Suzuki [9] showed that different bands were produced when using rabbit antisera reacting to *Anisakis* larvae and *Ascaris suum* in immunoelectrophoresis of *Anisakis* larvae antigens. He then demonstrated that hemoglobin of *Anisakis* larvae was responsible for this and concluded that the majority of E-S antigens were made up of hemoglobin. Asaishi [10] developed a rabbit antiserum reacting to *Anisakis* larvae hemoglobin and showed immunohistologically that this antibody reacted only to the perienteric cavity and not to the other organelles, including the Renette cells of *Anisakis* larvae. The antiserum did not react with *Ascaris suum*. *Anisakis* hemoglobin has been thought to be very specific to the larvae, but it also reacted to *Pseudoterranova decipiens* larvae. The antigens which were detected by monoclonal antibodies described in this chapter seem to be different from hemoglobins of *Anisakis* larvae becase: (a) the localization of antigens was different in *Anisakis* larvae; and (b) the antigens were specific to

Anisakis larvae and did not cross-react with *Pseudoterranova decipiens* larvae. These monoclonal antibodies were suitable not only for the taxonomic identification of *Anisakis* larvae but also in the biochemical analysis of specific antigens of the larvae.

Using rabbit anti-*Anisakis* antiserum immunized with E-S antigens, Matthews [11] reported that the antigens contained proteolytic activity with trypsin-like properties and identified the major source as the esophageal glands. Ruitenberg [12] demonstrated considerable enzymic activity within the "excretory" cell (i.e., the Renette cells) and proposed that the system was secretory. In the immunofluorescent study using monoclonal antibodies, An2 and An6 reacted to both the Renette cells and intestine of the larvae, and they were also reactive to E-S antigens using ELISA. These results suggest that Renette cells may be involved in the production of E-S antigens. Further investigations using these monoclonal antibodies are necessary to elucidate the origin and pathogenetic properties of E-S antigens.

Collectively, these monoclonal antibodies appear to be useful in identifying the specific antigens of anisakid larvae and characterizing etiological aspects in anisakiasis. Furthermore, it is indicated that the high specificity of these antibodies can be applied in the serodiagnosis of patients with anisakiasis.

Intradermal Reaction

A considerable number of immunodiagnostic methods are available for anisakiasis. The intradermal reaction using extracts of *Anisakis* larvae is one. In preliminary screening using crude extracts of *Anisakis* larvae, intradermal reactions showed false-positive changes in controls free of anisakiasis, resulting in a low diagnostic value [13]. Suzuki et al. [14] reported on intradermal tests using hemoglobin from *Anisakis* larvae, with the result that hemoglobin of *Anisakis* larvae was made available as a screening test for the detection of antiserum against the worm. Nishino [15] also reported the results of skin tests using the antigen, concluding that a high titration of antiserum against *Anisakis* larvae was observed in normal subjects living in coastal areas; these results are suggestive of a preimmunizing state against *Anisakis* larvae. The results correlate well with the results of indirect hemagglutinin tests.

Sarles' Phenomenon

Several investigations have been carried out to detect the reactivity of antiserum against *Anisakis* larvae with the purpose of finding a complementary tool in the diagnosis of anisakiasis. Sarles' phenomenon is an immunological reaction against helminths and was first reported by Taliaferro and Sarles [16]. They showed that antiserum against *Nippostrongylus muris* and its larva made immunoprecipitates around the body, especially the oral and anal openings. This implies that antiserum is reactive to liquid antigens, so-called excretory/secretory antigens. These facts were confirmed by the use of *Anisakis* larvae and rabbit antiserum by Morishita and Nishimura [17]. They showed that these immunoprecipitates suppressed sloughing of the larvae. There have been reports of

Sarles' phenomenon in human cases of anisakiasis. In experimental anisakiasis of rabbits, Hayasaka et al. [18] concluded that incubating the immune sera with the larvae for 12 h and using the sera at a dilution of 1 : 16 was optimal for testing for Sarles' phenomenon. This protocol excludes possibility of false-positive reactions, which may give similar results to other diseases, including ascariasis and bronchial asthma. From the results of these experiments, Sarles' phenomenon is valuable in the diagnosis of anisakiasis as a complementary immunological test.

References

1. Kohler G, Milstein C (1975) Continuous cultures of fused cells secreting antibodies of predefined specificity. Nature 256: 495–497
2. Takahashi S, Sato N, Sato T, Takami T, Mukaiya M, Yagihashi A, Tsurushiin M, Hayasaka H, Kikuchi K, Ishikura H (1986) Detection of anti-*Anisakis* larvae antibodies using micro-ELISA method. Igakunoayumi 136: 691–692
3. Danforth HD (1982) Development of hybridoma-produced antibodies directed against *Eimeria tenella* and *E. mitis*. J Parasitol 68: 392–397
4. De Ibarra AAL (1982) Monoclonal antibodies to *Leishmania tropica major* : specificities and antigen location. Parasitology 85: 523–531
5. Gowe JS (1983) All metacyclic variable antigen types of *Trypanosoma conglence* identified using monoclonal antibodies. Nature 306: 389–391
6. Ortega-Pierres G (1984) Protection against *Trichinella spiralis* induced by a monoclonal antibody that promotes killing of newborn larvae by granulocytes. Parasit Immunol 6: 275–284
7. Epstein N (1981) Monoclonal antibodies against a specific surface determinants on malarial (*Plasmodium knowlesi*) merzoites block erythrocyte invasion. J Immunol 127: 212–217
8. Agatsuma T (1981) Electrophoretic studies on glucosephosphatase isomerase and phosphoglucomutase in two types of *Anisakis* larvae. Int J Parasitol 12: 35–39
9. Suzuki T (1968) Immunodiagnositic studies on anisakiasis. Jpn J Parasitol 17: 213–220
10. Asaishi K (1974) Antigenic analysis of *Anisakis* larva and application of fluorescent antibody technique to histological diagnosis of anisakiasis. Sapporo Med J 43: 104–120
11. Matthews B (1984) The source, release and specificity of proteolytic enzyme activity produced by *Anisakis simplex* larvae in vitro. J Helminth 58: 175–185
12. Ruitenberg EJ (1971)Histochemical properties of the excretory organ of *Anisakis sp.* larva. J Parasitol 6: 9–13
13. Hayasaka H, Ishikura H, Miyagi H, Ueno T, Utsumi A, Sato Y (1968) Immunological study on anisakiasis (1) on its intracutaneous reaction. J Jpn Soc Clin Surg 29: 81–87 (in Japanese)
14. Suzuki T, Shiraki T, Sekino S, Osturu M (1970) Studies on the immunological diagnosis of anisakiasis 3 intradermal test with purified antigen. Jpn J Parasitol 19: 1–9 (in Japanese)
15. Nishino T (1977) Epidemiological studies on anisakiasis. Sapporo Med J 46: 73–88 (in Japanese)
16. Taliaferro WH, Sarles MP (1939) The cellular reaction in skin, lungs and intestine of normal and immune rats after infection with *Nippostrongyrus muris*. J Infect Dis 64: 157–192
17. Morishita Y, Nishimura T (1968) Sarles phenomenon on *Anisakis* larvae. Jpn J Parasitol 17: 30 (in Japanese)
18. Hayasaka H, Mizugaki H, Asaishi K, Takagi R, Iwano H, Ishikura H, Aizawa M (1970) Immunological reaction of intestinal anisakiasis—especially on Sarles phenomenon. Minophagen Med Review 15: 54–58 (in Japanese)

Biopsy of Gastric Anisakiasis with Acute Symptoms

Y. Yazaki and M. Namiki

Introduction

Almost all cases of gastric anisakiasis with acute symptoms have been easily cured by endoscopic removal of the worm which penetrated the stomach wall without the need for surgical operation [1–8]. Therefore, pathological studies [9] of the stomach during the acute phase of gastric anisakiasis are very rare. In animal experiments, the main lesion of this disease is found in the submucosal part of the stomach, causing severe edema and eosinophilic cell infiltration around the penetrating worm [10]. In this chapter, biopsy findings of this disease are presented.

Subjects and Method

One to three biopsies at the site of larval penetration and other lesions, such as erosion, severe edema, and redness, were performed after endoscopic removal of the worm in nine cases (seven due to *Anisakis simplex* larva, two due to *Pseudoterranova decipiens* larva. The biopsied specimens were fixed in 10% formalin, embedded in paraffin, and processed for H and E staining in the conventional manner. The worms were removed from the stomach with biopsy forceps and identified parasitologically.

Results

Endoscopic and light-microscopic findings are summarized in Table 1. Histologically, only one case had normal gastric mucosa at the site of penetration, whereas the others showed abnormal findings such as edema and inflammatory cell infiltration.

The mucosa showed strong inflammatory cell infiltration with a notable amount of eosinophils in one 24-year-old male (case 6; Fig. 1). In case 7, a 36-year-old male whose endoscopic examination showed severe edema and redness on the gastric body, the biopsied specimen from the site of penetration and other sites showed severe inflammatory cell infiltration but no eosinophils.

Table 1. Comparison between endoscopic findings and histopathologic features by mucosa biopsy on gastric anisakiasis with acute symptoms

Case No.	Age, Sex	Site of penetration (No.of worm)	Endoscopic findings of penetration area	Histopathologic findings of mucosal biopsy
1	55, M	Upper posterior wall of stomach body A (1)	Edema	Slight inflamatory cell infiltration
2	47, F	Upper posterior wall of stomach body A (1)	Edema	Normal mucosa
3	25, M	Fornix A (1)	Redness	Submucosal edema and breeding
4	36, M	Pyrolus A (1)	Redness	Slight inflamatory cell infiltration
5	38, M	Pyrolus A (2)	Edema	Mucosal edema
6	24, M	Greater curvature of middle stomach body A (2)	Edema	Severe inflamatory cell infiltration with eosinophils
7	36, M	Greater curvature of lower stomach body A (1)	Edema Redness	Severe inflamatory cell infiltration with submucosal edema
8	27, M	Greater curvature of middle stomach body T (2)	Almost normal mucosa	Submucosal edema
9	30, M	Greater curvature of middle stomach body T (1)	Almost normal mucosa	Submucosal edema

A,Anisakis simplex larva; *T,Pseudoterranova decipiens* larva

Discussion

The pathogenesis of gastric anisakiasis with acute symptoms (due to *Anisakis simplex* larva or *Pseudoterranova decipiens* larva) is thought to be an immunoreaction induced by secondary infection. This allergic reaction is composed of an anaphylactic one, which causes a strong spasm of the stomach, and an Arthus reaction around the penetrating worm [10]. In animal experiments, these lesions have been mainly found in the submucosal part. In animal experiments, Nagano et al. [11] found fibrinoid necrosis, erosion, severe eosinophilic infiltration (with some lymphoid cells and neutrophils), edema, bleeding, and teleangiectasis of the capillaries in the gastric mucosa at the site of penetration by the worm. However, they did not observe such lesions in endoscopic biopsies in human cases. Nagano et al. only noted one case displaying severe eosinophilic

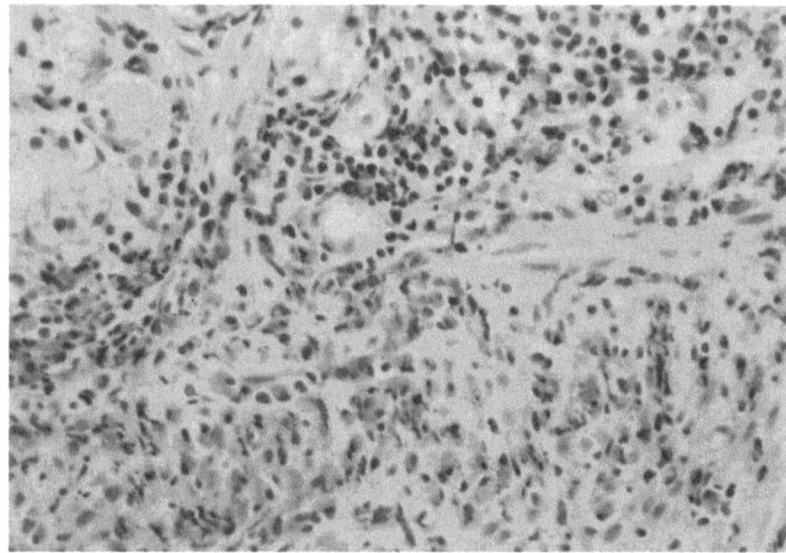

Fig. 1. Histopathological findings of the biopsied specimen. Microscopic examination revealed slight edema in the submucosa and eosinophilic cell infiltration in mucosa and submucosa. H.E. Staining, ×400

cell infiltration in the biopsy specimen at the site of penetration by the worm. Iwasaki and Toris [12] found an eosinophilic chemotactic factor in an *Anisakis* extract which caused infiltration of eosinophils around the penetrating worm without prior infecting by the *Anisakis* larva. However, this eosinophilic cell infiltration is restricted only to the area around the worm; it is not easy, therefore, to obtain this finding by endoscopic biopsy using small biopsy forceps in humans. In contrast, edema and nonspecific gastritis in the mucosal biopsy specimen are frequently found in this disease (44% each). These findings may represent the endoscopic findings of edema or redness of the gastric mucosa. It is believed that edema and gastritis are not specific but are very important histological findings in this disease.

Summary

One to three endoscopic biopsies were performed at the site of penetration and other parts of the stomach in nine cases of gastric anisakiasis wih acute symptoms (seven cases were due to *Anisakis simplex* larva, two cases to *Pseudoterranova decipiens* larva).

In one of the nine cases, severe eosinophilic cell infiltration was demonstrated in the biopsy specimen at the site of penetration by the worm.

Submucosal edema was found in 44% of the cases; inflamatory cell infiltration in four of the nine cases.

References

1. Namiki M, Morooka T, Kawauchi H, Veda N, Sekiya C, Nakagawa K (1969) On endoscopic observation of *Anisakis* larva in the stomach, and a few interesting findings. Gastroenterol Endosc 12 (abstract): 302 (in Japanese)
2. Namiki M, Morooka T, et al. (1970) Diagnosis of gastric anisakiasis with acute symptoms. Stomach Intestine 5: 1437–1440 (in Japanese)
3. Kawauchi H, Namiki M, Morooka T, Nakagawa K, Oguro T (1973) Gastric anisakiasis presenting acute gastrointestinal symptoms—with special reference to endoscopic and roentgenographic findings of *Anisakis* larva penetrating into the wall of the human stomach and to its clinical features. Stomach Intestine 8: 31–37 (in Japanese)
4. Doi K (1973) Clinical aspects of acute heterocheilidiasis of the stomach (due to larvae of *anisakis* and *terranova decipiens*)—Especially on its differential diagnosis by X-ray and endoscopy. Stomach Intestine 8: 1513–1518 (in Japanese)
5. Nagano K, Takagi K, Yanagawa K, Oishi O, Kagei K (1973) Acute heterocheilidiasis of the stomach (due to *Terranova decipiens*). Stomach Intestine 8: 81–85 (in Japanese)
6. Namiki M, Kawauchi H (1973): Anisakiasis. iagnosis Treatment 48: 1106–1112 (in Japanese)
7. Yazaki Y (1983) Gastric anisakiasis with acute symptoms in special reference to its diagnosis and treatment. Hokkaido J Med Sci 56: 362 (in Japanese)
8. Yazaki Y, Namiki M (1985) Gastric anisakiasis with acute symptoms—in special reference to its diagnostic imaging methods. Diagnostic Imaging Methods 5: 719–722 (in Japanese)
9. Okada K, Tsuchiya M, Tanaka K (1978) A case of acute anisakiasis of the stomach making rapid progress to parasitic granuloma. Progr Dig Endosc 12: 153–245 (in Japanese)
10. Suzuki T, Ishikawa H (1974) Pathogenic mechanisms, symptoms, and diagnosis of anisakiasis. Fishes and *Anisakis* (No. 7 Fisheries scientific series). Japanese Society of Fisheries, Koseishiya Koseikaku, Tokyo, pp 58–72 (in Japanese)
11. Nagano K, Sasaki Y, Ohtani N, Tokutomi Y, Nakaya S, Oishi K (1976) On biopsy of acute heterocheilidiasis of the stomach. Stomach Intestine 11: 195–201 (in Japanese)
12. Iwasaki K, Toris M (1982) Immunological profiles of anisakiasis—on new concept of pathogenesis of eosinophilic granuloma. Saishin Igaku 37: 1179–1185 (in Japanese)

Pathology of Gastric Anisakiasis

Y. Kikuchi, H. Ishikura, K. Kikuchi, and H. Hayasaka

Anisakiasis of the alimentary tract is divided into two types—gastric and intestinal anisakiasis. There are clear differences in the clinical and pathological findings between these two types. Van Thiel et al. [1] reported that most cases in the Netherlands were of the intestinal type. This was also found in the cases of the Iwanai district in Hokkaido, Japan [2]. By contrast, in the whole of Japan there were 167 reported gastric cases (76.7%) of the 218 cases of anisakiasis over a 5-year period (1969–1974) [3]. There are several clinical and pathological classifications of anisakiasis. Basically, the lesions found in anisakiasis are classified into two categories—fulminant and mild [4].

Fulminant Form

In Japan, the number of cases in the fulminant form of gastric anisakiasis that have been examined pathologically is very low compared with the number of cases of intestinal anisakiasis. As a result of advances in gastroendoscopic techniques, *Anisakis* larvae partly penetrating the gastric wall can be removed in this fulminant form. However, also because of these advances, we can no longer obtain surgical specimens of the fulminant form from the stomach wall.

Macroscopic Findings

Clinically, at the time of onset of this form, patients report epigastralgia, nausea, and vomiting. The condition is frequently misdiagnosed as acute gastritis or gastric ulcer. With the onset of symptoms, the *Anisakis simplex* larva may be observed by gastric endoscopy partly penetrating the wall of the stomach. On the mucosa itself, distinct edema and petechiae are provoked but to a lesser extent than is the case with the fulminant form of intestinal anisakiasis. Multiple spotted bleeding or small erosions are also found. It is suspected that migration of a larva gives rise to these lesions or, possibly, it is due to several larvae migrating to the stomach wall at the same time.

Microscopic Findings

The cut surface of an *Anisakis simplex* larva in the submucosal layer can be seen histopathologically. Even though *Anisakis* larvae are not found in any one area of the phlegmonous wall, they may occasionally be detected by searching over an area of several square centimeters. The larva is surrounded by intense thickening of the gastric wall; there is edema and massive eosinophilic infiltration of all layers with other cellular components, neutrophils, histiocytes, and lymphocytes. The larva is usually intact and clearly visible in this form. In this lesion, angitis and fibrinous exudation may occur. Although the lesion of the fulminant form of gastric anisakiasis is usually milder than in intestinal anisakiasis, the fulminant form conforms with the phlegmonous reaction as classified by Kojima et al. [5]. However, in unsensitized rabbits injected intradermally with the cultured supernatant of living larvae, marked edema, hemorrhage, and a cell reaction, including eosinophils, appeared [5]. This phenomenon shows that metabolic products of living larvae as secretions or excretions can provoke a phlegmonous reaction in unsensitized rabbits. This reaction is most intensive when animals are injected with a cultured supernatant of molting larvae. This phenomenon might explain the phlegmonous reaction of anisakiasis by primary infection or penetration of the larvae itself through the digestive tract. Van Thiel et al. [1] and Kuipers [6] reported the phlegmonous lesion of intestinal anisakiasis to be local hypersensitivity. They considered that secondary infection by *Anisakis* larvae would cause eosinophilic phlegmon on the gastrointestinal wall close to the area of the primary larval infection (double-hit theory). The mechanism of the accumulation of eosinophils around the *Anisaksi* larva has not yet been clarified. Recently, Torisu et al. [7] reported that the *Anisakis* larva has a potent chemotactic factor selectively for eosinophils and termed it eosinophilic chemotactic factor derived from parasite (ECF-P). ECF-P was detected in the aqueous extract and also in the culture supernatant of *Anisakis* larvae; it is heat labile and has a molecular weight of 40 000. Thus, the mechanisms of provoked eosinophilia may be separated from Arthus-type reaction in the lesion of Anisakiasis.

There have been many experimental studies by Japanese investigators which substantiate these pathological findings.

Anisakiasis has been experimentally induced in rabbits [5, 8, 9] and guinea pigs [9] by the injection of live *Anisakis* larvae or a homogenate of the larvae intraperitoneally or subcutaneously. To provoke an Arthus-type reaction by secondary antigen injection, live *Anisakis* larvae were introduced orally or operatively into the stomach wall or subcutaneous tissue of rabbits. The second exposure of *Anisakis* antigens in the primed hosts resulted in an intensive phlegmonous reaction similar to the Arthus-type reaction with eosinophils, in contrast to unsensitized control animals. Abscess formation around the larvae was frequently found. Conversely, in primary sensitization, live larvae were given orally, and then a second exposure with a larval homogenate was injected into the stomach wall of the animals. The pathological findings of the stomach wall of primed animals showed wide abscess formation with marked eosinophilic infiltration around the injected homogenate. In the unsensitized control animals, a small abscess without edema and reactive cells after 7 days of homogenate injection could be observed.

Table 1. Frequency of stomach and intestinal anisakiasis in pathological classification

Histological type	Kojima et al. [5]		Shiraki [10]		Iwano et al. [3]	
	Stomach	Intest.	Stomach	Intest.	Stomach	Intest.
Phlegmon	0	5	6	8	6	16
Abscess	10	7	20	7	7	1
Abscess-granuloma	3	4	9	1	22	3
Granuloma	0	0	2	4	/	/
Total	13	16	37	20	35	20

Table 2. Location of anisakiasis in the stomach

Location in stomach	Ishikura (1967)	Iwano et al. [3]	Total
Cardia	2	2	4
Angle	10	17	27
Fundus	78	55	133
Prepyloric	32	12	44
Pyloric	29	8	37
Greater curvature	29	29	58
Lesser curvature	19	10	56
Anterior wall	35	21	56
Posterior wall	29	39	68

Mild Form

Patients in this category of anisakiasis may complain of gastralgia, loss of appetite, and an epigastric tumor, which may be misdiagnosed as stomach cancer or stomach ulcer. Cases of the mild form of gastric anisakiasis have been examined pathologically much more frequently than cases of the fulminant form in Japan. Kojima et al. [5] found 13 cases of the mild form, Shiraki [10] found a total of 37, and Iwano et al. [3] reported 29 cases of the mild form of a total of 35 cases (Table 1). More than 3700 cases of this form have been reported following these studies.

Macroscopic Findings

The location of the migrating larva in the stomach, as shown in Table 2, is most frequently at the fundus, posterior wall, and greater major curvature [11]. In the affected area, localized induration, a small ulcer, and erosion are observed and are sometimes misdiagnosed as stomach cancer or stomach ulcer. When penetrated by the larvae, the stomach becomes densely scarred at the serosa or indurated by the adhesion of the major omentum. These tumorous lesions may be induced by the pathological allergic reaction, as previously explained, or parasitic granuloma caused by the prolonged presence of *Anisakis* larva in the gastric wall.

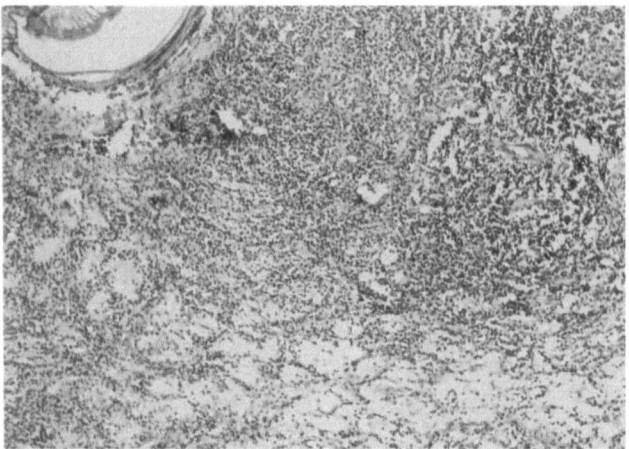

Fig. 1. Phlegmon-formation type. In the *upper left*, cut surface of fresh *Anisakis simplex* larva surrounded by massive neutrophils and eosinophils as seen in the submucosa of the stomach wall

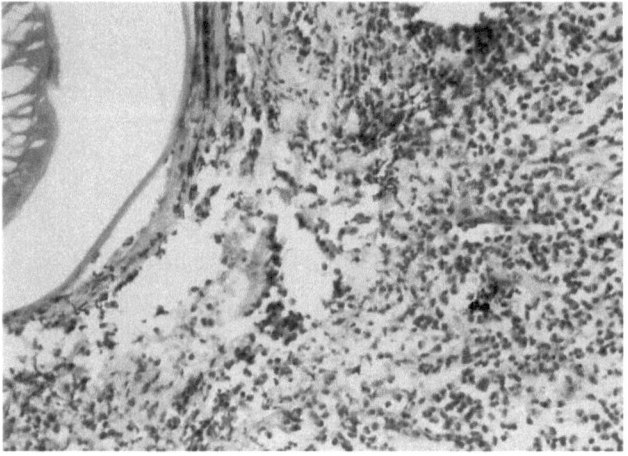

Fig. 2. Higher magnification of Fig. 1

Microscopic Findings

The pathological classification of anisakiasis has been described by Kojima et al. [5].

First stadium—phlegmon-formation type of Arthus reaction. This type is more frequently observed in intestinal anisakiasis than in gastric anisakiasis (Figs. 1, 2). It is almost the same as the fulminant form of anisakiasis and its pathological findings are described in detail in the section dealing with the fulminant form above.

Second stadium—abscess-formation type. Most cases arise from acute or chronic gastric anisakiasis. A marked abscess with many eosinophils, histiocytes, and lymphocytes is observed around the slightly degenerating larva or its debris (Figs. 3–11). The degenerating larva is surrounded by intense necrotic tissue at the inner layer of the granuloma with infiltration of eosinophils into the larva. A small amount of granulomatous tissue surrounding the abscess is infiltrated by eosinophils, histiocytes, and lymphocytes with edema and fibrin exudation or fibrinoid degeneation. In their experiments, Kojima et al. [5] called this type of reaction an "excervation" reaction. Their experiments showed that this phleg-monous reaction resulted from exposure of the parasitic antigen, especially excreted material, secretions, or visceral antigens.

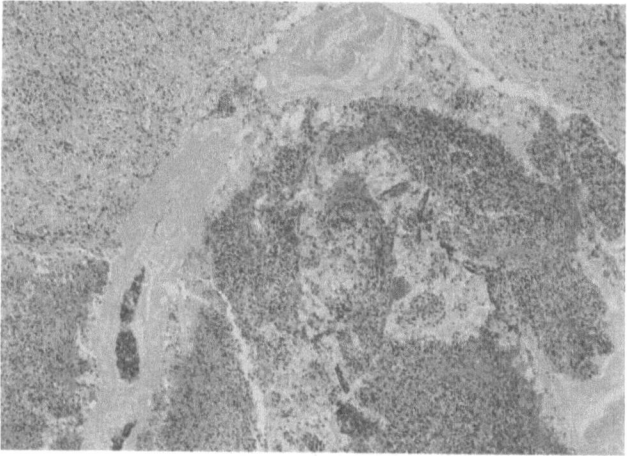

Fig. 3. Abscess-formation type. In the *center*, a markedly destroyed larval body is found infiltrated by massive neutrophils and eosinophils

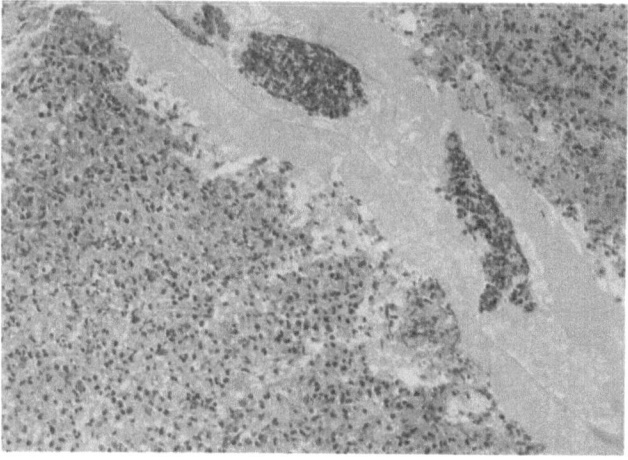

Fig. 4. Higher magnification of Fig. 3. Massive neutrophils and eosinophils are infiltrating the body of the larva

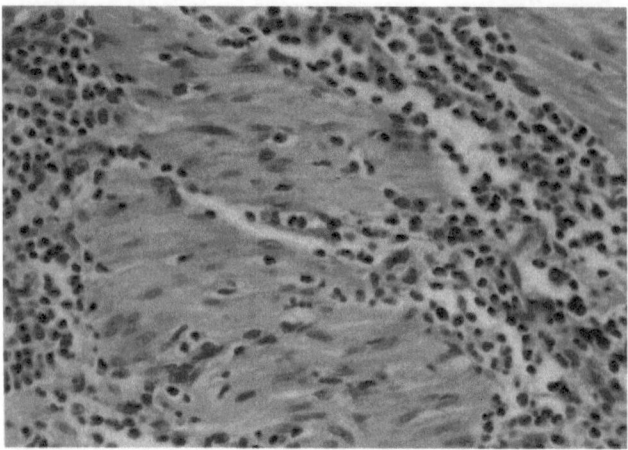

Fig. 5. Lamina muscularis propria of stomach wall in abscess-formation type. Marked eosinophils, neutrophils, and lymphocytes are found

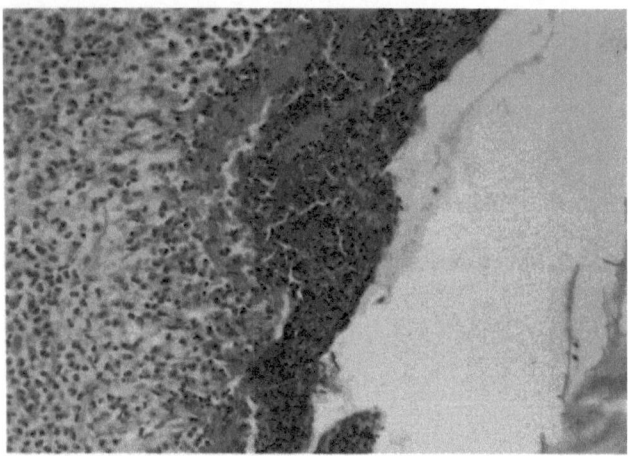

Fig. 6. Abscess-formation type showing signs of exacerbation. On the *right*, degenerated larva and markedly destroyed larval cuticula are seen with neutrophils and eosinophils

Third stadium—abscess granuloma-formation type. In cases of gastric anisa-kiasis, the abscess becomes reduced after more than 6 months from the time of larval infection (Figs. 12–14). Sometimes, a degenerating larva is found in the center of an abscess surrounded by granulation tissue. The reacting cell infiltration including eosinophils is less intensive than in the abscess-formation type. The degenerating larva is invaded by eosinophils and sometimes surrounded by foreign body giant cells. Lymphocyte infiltration may be dominant instead of eosinophils in this lesion.

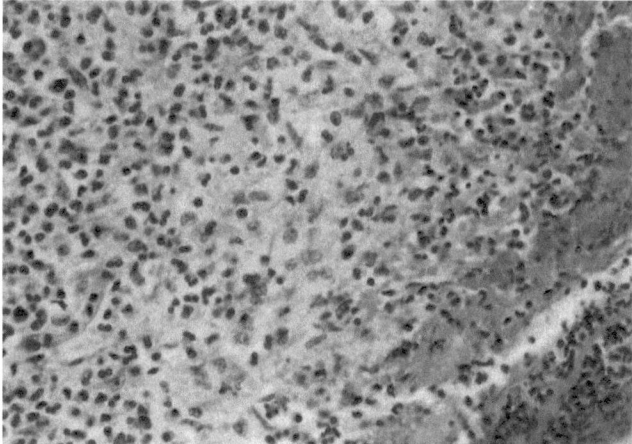

Fig. 7. Higher magnification of Fig. 6. Markedly infiltrated neutrophils, eosinophils, and histiocytes with destroyed larva

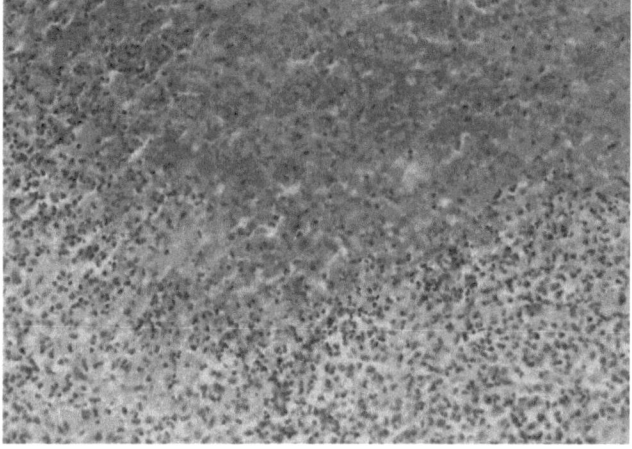

Fig. 8. Higher magnification of the exacerbated area of Fig. 6. In the *top right*, there is degenerated tissue surrounded by neutrophils, eosinophils, and histiocytes

Fourth stadium—granuloma-formation type. The most advanced stage of anisa-kiasis shows apparently larval debris surrounded by a small amount of abscess or granulomatous tissue with collagenization, foreign body giant cells, and mild eosinophilic infiltration. This type of lesion is occasionally observed in advanced and long-standing cases of gastric and intestinal anisakiasis. This may be why diagnosis of these lesions of chronic gastric anisakiasis is delayed.

Depending on the time following larval infection, destruction of the larva may progress systemically. Conversely, it is possible that the grade of larval destruc-tion may indicate the period of larval infection. However, these pathological stadia of anisakiasis are not strictly separated but form a continuum.

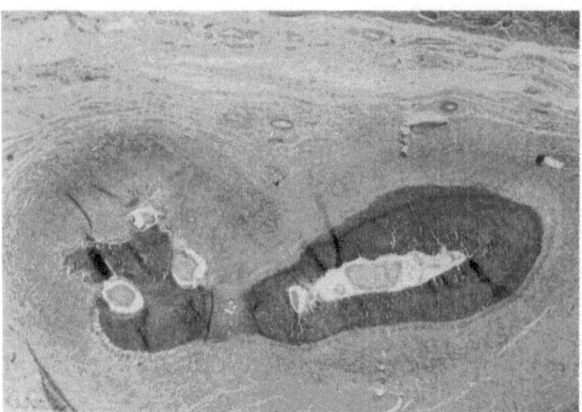

Fig. 9. Abscess-formation type with granulomatous change. In the center of the submucosal abscess, the degenerated larva (five cut surfaces) is surrounded by the abscess with signs of exacerbation, many foreign body giant cells, and fibrosis

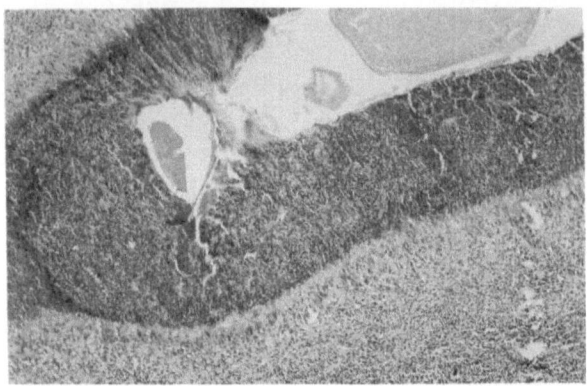

Fig. 10. Higher magnification of Fig. 9

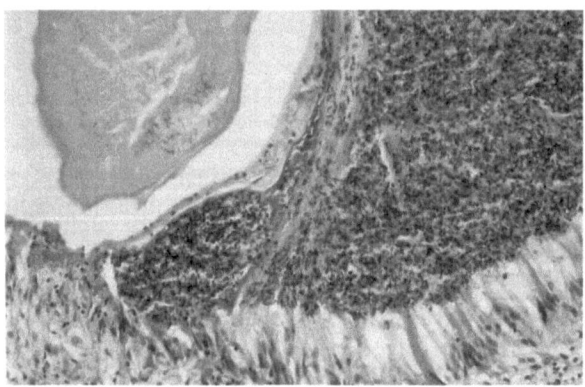

Fig. 11. Higher magnification of Fig. 9

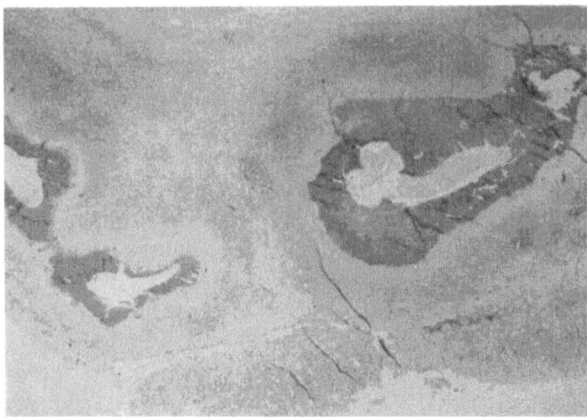

Fig. 12. Abscess granuloma-formation type. In the submucosa of the stomach, the degenerated larva (four cut surfaces) is surrounded by the abscess and granuloma with foreign body giant cells and fibroblast. If these findings are compared with those in Fig. 9, the exacerbation finding becomes one of low-grade cell infiltration

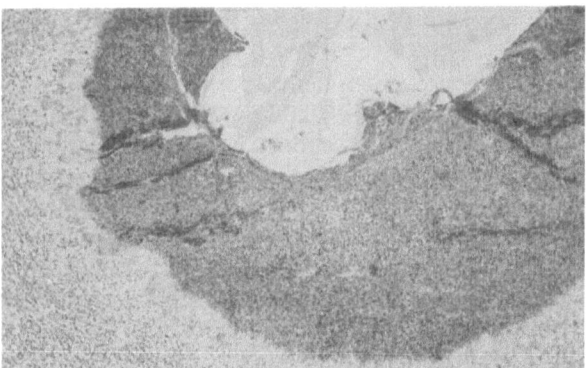

Fig. 13. Higher magnification of Fig. 12

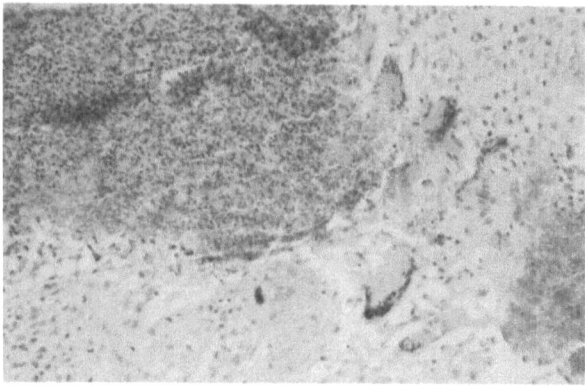

Fig. 14. Higher magnification of Fig. 12

Shiraki [10] compared the pathological characteristics of anisakiasis and the degree of preservation of the *Anisakis* larva itself. Of the four types of pathological classification [5], the best preservation of the larva is seen in the phlegmonous type, where it occasionally remains alive. In the lesion of the abscess type, the larva is found in the vital cuticula and/or muscle cells; in the lesions of the abscess-granulomatous type, intense degeneration of all components of the larva is indicated. This latter finding is the highest grade of degeneration of the larvae. By contrast, Saeki et al. [12] reported that destruction of the larvae approximately paralleled the degree of immune status of the rabbits that were subcutaneously and intramurally immunized with them. From these results, they concluded that immunity was closely related to the host reactivity and degeneration of parasitic bodies.

These histopathological observations show the antigen-antibody reaction to be anaphylaxis, Arthus-type, and delayed-type reaction caused by the host-parasite interaction.

Recently, most available reports on immunological studies investigating the pathogenesis of anisakiasis have come from the humoral antibody response of rabbits and guinea pigs.

Taniguchi [13] and Kikuchi et al. [14] reported that immunized rabbits or guinea pigs with PBS extract or live *Anisakis* larvae showed passive cutaneous anaphylaxis (PCA) positively for a period of 10 days. On the possible relation between IgE and experimental anisakiasis, Kobayashi et al. [15] and Sato et al. [16] have reported in vivo and in vitro studies using guinea pigs.

Although numerous reports on humoral immunity are available, only a few investigations have been made on cellular immunity in anisakiasis. Kikuchi et al. [8] reported on intracutaneous reactions in rabbits, which indicated an immediate reaction by supernatants and a delayed reaction by a precipitate of a PBS extraction of *Anisakis* larvae. On the other hand, Saeki [9] reported on the delayed-type reaction in anisakiasis. In that study, the delayed-type cutaneous reaction in vivo and the migration-inhibition (MI) test in vitro were used to analyze the cell-mediated immunity in experimental anisakiasis using guinea pigs and rabbits. The delayed-type reaction was shown by a marked skin reaction in sensitized guinea pigs but not in sensitized rabbits. Further investigations are necessary to clarify whether this is due to a species difference. On the other hand, the MI test proved to be more sensitive than the skin reaction in showing the existence of a delayed-type reaction in sensitized animals. With the MI test, it is suggested that experimental anisakiasis shows a delayed-type reaction in the host infected with *Anisakis* larvae. This report of Saeki is the first to show in vitro cell-mediated immunity to anisakiasis.

References

1. Van Thiel PH, Kuipers FC, Roskam TH (1960) A nematode parasitic to herring, causing acute abdominal syndromes in man. Trop Geogr Med 12: 97–113
2. Ishikura H, Kikuchi Y, Hayasaka H, Miyagi H, Ueno T (1968) Anisakiasis in Hokkaido. Jpn J Clin Surg 29: 49–60 (in Japanese)
3. Iwano H, Ishikura H, Hayasaka H (1974) Statistical observation of anisakiasis in Japan for the last 5 years. Geka Shinryo 16: 1336–1342 (in Japanese)

4. Suzuki T (1968) Studies on the immunological diagnosis of anisakiasis: I. Antigenic analysis of *Anisakis* larvae by means of electrophoresis. Jpn J Parasitol 17: 213–220 (in Japanese)
5. Kojima K, Koyanagi T, Shiraki K (1966) Pathological studies of anisakiasis (parasitic abscess formation in gastrointestinal tracts). Jpn J Clin Med 24: 134–143 (in Japanese)
6. Kuipers FC (1964) Pathogenese van de haringwarmflegmone bij de mens. Nederlands Tijdschrift Geneeskunde 108: 304–305
7. Torisu M, Iwasaki K, Tanaka J, Iino H, Yoshida T (1983) *Anisakis* and eosinophil: Pathogenesis and biologic significance of eosinophilic phlegmon in human anisakiasis. In: Yoshida T, Toris M (eds) Immunology of the eosinophil. Elsevier, New York, pp 343–367
8. Kikuchi Y, Ueda T, Yoshiki T, Aizawa M, Ishikura H (1967) Experimental immunopathological studies of intestinal anisakiasis. Igaku No Ayumi 62: 731–736 (in Japanese)
9. Saeki H (1975) Studies on cell-mediated immunity in experimental anisakiasis. J Sapporo Medical College 44: 309–322 (in Japanese)
10. Shiraki T (1969) On the pathological diagnosis of gastrointestinal larva migrans (on anisakiasis). Saishin-igaku 24: 378–389 (in Japanese)
11. Ishikura H (1969) Occurrence of anisakiasis and its clinical presentation. Saishin-igaku 24: 357–365 (in Japanese)
12. Saeki H, Mizugaki H, Ishikura H, Hayasaka H (1972) Immunological studies on anisakiasis: II. Participation of immune response in host-tissue reaction and destruction of parasite bodies. Hokkaido J Med Sci 47: 541–550 (in Japanese)
13. Taniguchi M (1970) Homocytotropic antibody of rabbits, sensitized or infected with *Anisakis* (Nematoda). Jpn J Parasitol 19: 189–195 (in Japanese)
14. Kikuchi K, Toyokawa O, Nakamura K, Ishiyama H, Yokota H, Sato H, Natori T, Ishikura H, Aizawa M (1970) Immunopathology of experimental anisakiasis. Minophagen Medical Review 15: 54–58 (in Japanese)
15. Kobayashi A, Watanabe N, Endo T (1974) Suppression of immunological mast cell degranulation to bovine serum albumin in mice following *Anisakis* infection. (Abstract) Proceedings of the 3rd International Congress of Parasitology Munich, Aug. 25–31, 1974. FACTA Publication, Vienna, pp 1075–1076
16. Sato Y, Yamashita T, Otsuru M, Suzuki T (1975) Studies on the aetiology of anisakiasis. I. The anaphylactic reaction of digestive tract to the worm extracts. Jpn J Parasitol 24: 192–202 (in Japanese)

Treatment of Gastric Anisakiasis with Acute Symptoms

M. NAMIKI and Y. YAZAKI

The symptoms of acute gastric anisakiasis diminish immediately after endoscopic removal of the larva [1–7]. This is the only means of treating the disease at present.

If removal of the larva is attempted, it is important not to try and take the larva itself; the larva and the surrounding gastric mucosa should be removed simultaneously by biopsy forceps. In this way, separation of the larva body, leaving the head behind in the gastric mucosa, can be prevented (Fig. 1). When the larva has been detached from the gastric mucosa, the biopsy forceps are straightened, the larva is gradually pulled into the channel of the endoscope, and then out of then endoscope through the channel. The larva can be taken alive by removing the metal holder and rubber cap at the opening of the biopsy forceps. After removal of one larva, it is important to make a close and careful inspection of the entire gastric mucosa before removing the endoscope. We have often observed multiple larva contagion. The symptoms of the disease, such as epigastralgia, nausea, and vomiting, will not disappear if another larva remains in the stomach. We have experience of a patient with as many as four larvae in the gastric mucosa at the same time.

If the symptoms do not improve after removal of larva, as stated, multiple contagion should be suspected and careful endoscopic examination of the stomach, duodenum, and esophagus performed immediately. It is necessary to keep in mind that *Anisakis* larvae can invade any part of the gastrointestinal tract.

One experimental report suggests that the larva moving through the gastrointestinal tract can be killed by pyrantel pamoate [8]. But once the larva penetrates the gastrointestinal wall, even if the larva is dead, it will remain there as an antigen-developing eosinophilic granuloma (Fig. 2) [9].

Removed larvae should be fixed in alcohol or formalin and sent to an institute where they can be precisely identified. There is always the possibility that a new type of contagion may be found. Treatment itself accompanies the diagnosis in this disease.

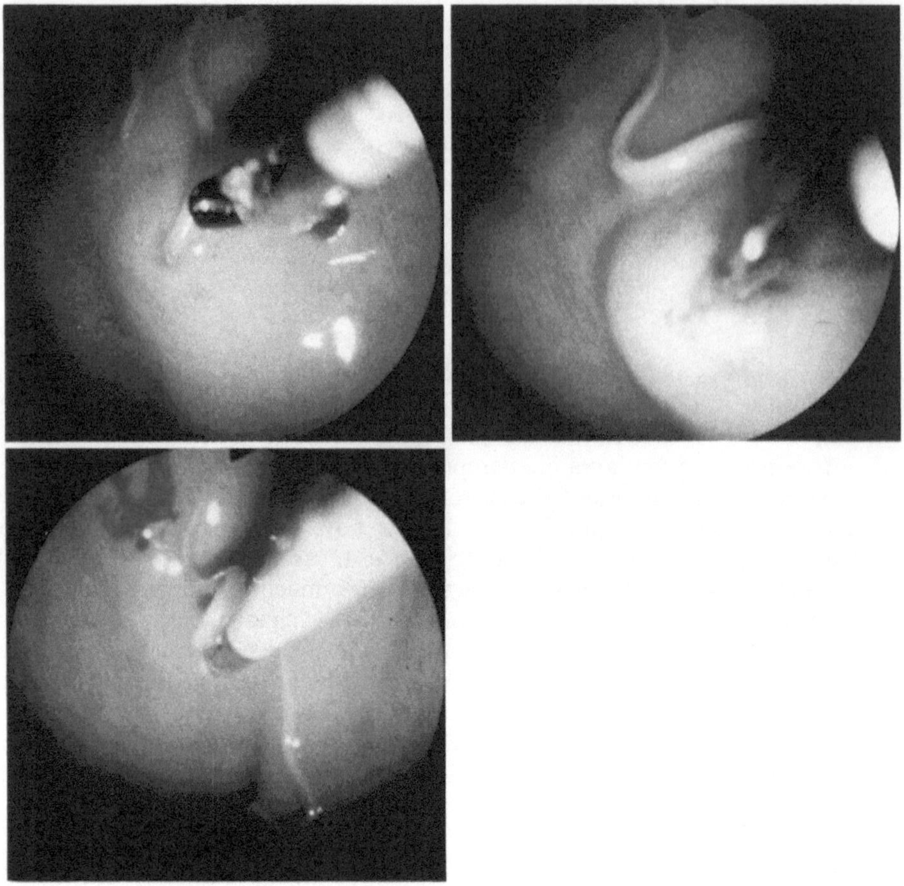

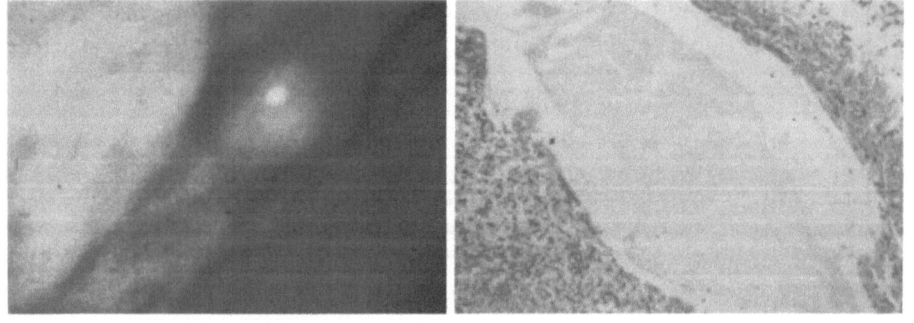

Fig. 1a–c. Endoscopic removal by biopsy forceps of *Anisakis simplex* larva that has penetrated gastric mucosa

Fig. 2. a Gastrofiberscopic findings of eosinophilic granuloma of the stomach. **b** Histological findings of resected gastric eosinophilic granuloma, showing *Anisakis simplex* larva and severe infiltration by eosinophils. H.E. Staining, ×200

References

1. Namiki M, Morooka T, Kawauchi H, Ueda N, Sekiya C, Nakagawa K, Furuta T, Oguro T, Kamada H (1970) Diagnosis of gastric anisakiasis with acute symptoms. Stomach Intestine 5: 1437–1440 (in Japanese)
2. Kawauchi H, Namiki M, Morooka T, Nakagawa K, Oguro T (1973) Gastric anisakiasis presenting acute gastrointestinal symptoms—with special reference to endoscopic and roentgenographic findings of *Anisakis* larva penetrating into the wall of the human stomach and to its clinical features. Stomach Intestine 8: 31–37 (in Japanese)
3. Doi K (1973) Clinical aspects of acute Heterocheilidiasis of the stomach. (Due to larvae of *Anisakis* and *Terranova decipiens*) Especially on its differential diagnosis by X-ray and endoscopy. Stomach Intestine 8: 1513–1518 (in Japanese)
4. Nagano K, Takagi K, Yanagawa K, Ohishi K, Kagei N(1973) Acute Heterocheilidiasis of the stomach (due to *Terranova decipiens*). Stomach Intestine 8: 81–85 (in Japanese)
5. Masayoshi Namiki, Hideki Kawauchi (1973) Anisakiasis. Diagnosis and treatment 48: 1106–1112 (in Japanese)
6. Yazaki Y (1983) Gastric anisakiasis with acute symptoms in special reference to its diagnosis and treatment: Hokkaido J Med Sci 56: 362 (in Japanese)
7. Yazaki Y, Namiki M (1985) Gastric anisakiasis with acute symptoms—in special reference to its diagnostic imaging methods. Diag Imag Meth 5: 719–722 (in Japanese)
8. Iwano H, Ishikura H, Hayasaka A (1973) A study on prophylaxis of anisakiasis: III. Effect of the pyrantel pamoate. Hokkaido J Surg 19: 83–90 (in Japanese)
9. Okada K, Tsuchiya M, Tanaka N, Hashizume Y (1978) A case of acute anisakiasis of the stomach making rapid progress to parasitic granuloma. Progr Dig Endosc 12: 153–245 (in Japanese)

Gastric Terranovasis

K. Nagano

Distribution

In 1972, working independently, our group [1, 2] in Hakodate and the group of Suzuki et al. [3] in Asahikawa, Hokkaido, using endoscopes removed living *Pseudoterranova decipiens* larvae that had penetrated the gastric mucosa of patients with acute gastric symptoms. These were the first reported discoveries of *Pseudoterranova decipiens* larva parasitism in humans. Since then, reported cases of visceral migration of *Pseudoterranova decipiens* larvae (so-called terranovasis) have increased in number.

The characteristics of the mode of occurrence of terranovasis are described below.

Occurrence by Organ

Documented cases of terranovasis have only involved the stomach. There have been no reported occurrences in the intestine. It is generally believed that no difference exists between *Anisakis* and *Terranova* group larvae in the survival rate in physiological saline at room temperature. There was no difference between the two types of larva in the resistance to 0.3% hydrochloride solution and the penetrating ratio of 1% agar gel; this was also the case in experiments using orally administered living larvae in rabbits [4–6]. Terranovasis in the intestine has not been reported as yet. In gastric terranovasis, a fulminant form, presenting severe gastric symptoms, is predominant, while a mild form, which mimics eosinophilic granuloma, is extremely rare or nonexistent [7]; thus, the fulminant form is discussed here.

Occurrence by Region

In Japan, gastric terranovasis is diagnosed frequently in the northern regions (very often on the northernmost island, Hokkaido, and Aomori prefecture on the northern tip of Honshu, the largest of the Japanese islands) and very rarely or not at all in the southern part of Japan.

According to a nationwide survey that Koyama et al. [8] conducted by questionnaire of 1242 anisakiasis patients, 1045 (73.4%) were caused by *Anisakis simplex* larvae, 160 (11.2%) by *Pseudoterranova decipiens* larvae, and 219

Table 1. Statistical classification of larvae causing human anisakiasis in Japan

Region	*Anisakis simplex*		*Pseudoterranova decipiens*		Unknown		
	No. of cases	Percent	No. of cases	Percent	No. of cases	Percent	Total No. of cases
Hokkaido	442	(69.9)	138	(21.8)	52	(8.2)	632
Tohoku	4	(7.8)	0		47	(92.2)	51
Kanto	30	(90.9)	1	(3.0)	2	(6.1)	33
Chubu	164	(68.3)	19	(7.9)	57	(23.8)	240
Kinki	178	(98.3)	1	(0.6)	2	(1.1)	181
Chugoku	21	(63.6)	0		12	(36.4)	33
Shikoku	14	(87.5)	0		2	(12.5)	16
Kyushu	191	(80.6)	1	(0.4)	45	(19.0)	237
Okinawa	1	(100)	0		0		1
Total	1045	(73.4)	160	(11.2)	219	(15.4)	1424

After Koyama et al. [8]

(15.4%) by unknown larvae; thus, the ratio of cases caused by *Pseudoterranova decipiens* larvae is relatively large (Table 1). The survey also reports that in the Hokkaido and Chubu regions, especially in Ishikawa prefecture, where anisakiasis is common, anisakiasis due to *Pseudoterranova decipiens* larvae is frequently found, but few cases are found in the Kinki region and further south. On the other hand, in the Kushu region where anisakiasis is also found at a high frequency, only one case of anisakiasis due to *Pseudoterranova decipiens* larvae was found. According to a similar survey by Ishikura published at about the same time as the survey of Koyama et al. [8] of 1859 anisakiasis cases, 1755 cases (94.4%) were caused by *Anisakis simplex* larvae and 68 cases (3.7%) by *Pseudoterranova decipiens* larvae, and 36 cases (1.9%) by unknown larvae (Table 2). Of 1649 cases of anisakiasis reported at the 27th Congress of the Japan Gastroenterological Endoscopy (May 1984),1639 cases of gastric anisakiasis with acute symptoms were studied [9]. Substantially in agreement with the Ishikura report (Table 2), 1515 cases (92.4%) were ascribed to *Anisakis simplex* larvae, 78 (4.8%) to *Pseudoterranova decipiens* larvae, and 46 (2.8%) to unknown larvae. Of the 152 cases we experienced in 1984, 88 (57.9%) were caused by *Anisakis simplex* larvae, 53 (34.9%) by *Pseudoterranova decipiens* larvae, and 11 (7.2%) by unknown larvae (Table 3). Karasawa experienced 195 cases of gastric anisakiasis in Asahikawa [8]; in this group, 115 cases (59.3%) were due to *Anisakis simplex* larvae, 61 (31.4%) to *Pseudoterranova decipiens* larvae, and 18 (9.3%) to unknown larvae; these results are in good accord with our data (Table 3). Data for the whole of Japan show a lower ratio of *Pseudoterranova decipiens* larva since these figures include regions where the larva is seldom found. However, when all the data for Hokkaido are compiled, the ratio between *Anisakis simplex* and *Pseudoterranova decipiens* larvae turns out to be about 2:1, respectively. It is natural that the Koyama et al. report, which is strongly influenced by the Karasawa report, should show a high incidence of *Pseudoterranova decipiens* larvae.

Table 2. Statistical classification of larvae causing human anisakisis in Japan

Author	*Anisakis simplex* larva		*Pseudoterranova decipiens* larva		Unknown		Total No. of cases	Reference Literature
	No. of cases	Percent	No. of cases	Percent	No. of cases	Percent		
Nagano	1515	(92.4)	78	(4.8)	46	(2.8)	1639	[9]
Ishikura	1755	(94.4)	68	(3.7)	36	(1.9)	1859	[8]

Table 3. Statistical classification of larvae causing acute gastric anisakiasis in Hokkaido

District	*Anisakis simplex* larva		*Pseudoterranova decipiens* larva		Unknown		Total No. of cases	Reference Literature
	No. of cases	Percent	No. of cases	Percent	No. of cases	Percent		
Hokkaido	88	(57.9)	53	(34.9)	11	(7.2)	152	[9]
Asahi-kawa	115	(59.3)	61	(31.4)	18	(9.3)	195	[8]

Causes of Localization

A comparison between the Hokkaido and Kyushu islands reveals that, while in both areas anisakiasis is diagnosed in very high rates, terranovasis is relatively frequent only in Hokkaido and only 1 of 637 anisakiasis cases in Kyushu was due to *Pseudoterranova decipiens* larva. Kagei [10] reported that most of the hosts of *Anisakidae* larvae are fish and squids that wander generally around the northern Pacific Ocean; these animals become highly parasitized by *Anisakidae* larvae with changes in their dietary habits from single zooid plankton to other small fish and then to omnivorous eating patterns. Compiling many reports, Kagei found that while *Anisakis simplex* larva is found in 132 kinds of fish and one kind of squid inhabiting all the sea areas of Japan, *Pseudoterranova decipiens* larva is found only in a few kinds, including some flat fish (e.g., halibut), cod (e.g., Alaska pollack), sailfin sand fish, nurf smelt, and arctic smelt. Most of these fish are found in the seas around northern Japan and not in the sea around Kyushu. This difference in the distribution of host fish parasitized by the larvae is reflected in the difference in frequency and diagnosis of this disease in different geographical locations.

Rates of Discovery at Different Sites in One Region

Since 1970, when Namiki et al. [11] succeeded in the endoscopic removal of the larva, the number of cases of gastric anisakiasis has rapidly increased; the ratio of *Anisakis simplex* and *Pseudoterranova decipiens* larvae initially differed among various places in Hokkaido, but it has gradually tended to approach a ratio of 2:1. Despite many reports of anisakiasis in Hakodate, strangely enough

Table 4. Statistical classification of larvae causing acute gastric anisakiasis around
Tsugaru Strait

District	Anisakis simplex		Pseudoterranova decipiens		Unknown		Total No. of cases	Reference Literature
	No. of cases	Percent	No. of cases	Percent	No. of cases	Percent		
Aomori	14	(66.7)	7	(33.3)	—	—	21	[12]
Hirosaki	9	(60.0)	6	(40.0)	—	—	15	[13]
Hakodate	10	(71.4)	4	(28.6)	8	—	14	[14]

no reports of this condition have been reported in the northern part of the Tohoku region where fish from the same sea, including the Tsugaru Strait, are eaten.
It was only recently that reports of cases from this region were published. Table
4 summarizes the main reports [12, 13]. According to these, one characteristic of
gastric anisakiasis found in Aomori prefecture is a higher ratio of *Pseudoterranova decipiens* larvae. This agrees well with my own data reported in 1974 [14]
(Table 4). But here, as the number of cases increased, the ratio of terranovasis
to the total number of anisakiasis cases decreased and ultimately settled at the
level shown in Table 3. It is hard to believe that for the inhabitants of these two
areas, who share nearly identical customs and habits, a disease caused by fish
parasitized by *Anisakidae* larvae and caught in the same part of the sea has so
great a difference in frequency. It is to be expected that with time the regional
data for northern Tohoku and Hakodate will come to show similar ratios.

Symptoms and Clinical Diagnosis

There are no characteristic symptoms of anisakiasis caused by *Pseudoterranova
decipiens* larvae; they are very similar to those of anisakiasis due to *Anisakis
simplex* larvae [15–17]. The slight differences that may exist can be cited as follows.

Time of Occurrence

Anisakis simplex larva finds its host in a variety of fish in the seas close to Japan
and because the parasitized fish are caught throughout the year its occurrence is
similarly seen all year round and normally does not show a concentration in any
particular month. Conversely, in the case of *Pseudoterranova decipiens* larva,
there are very few kinds of host fish and the disease frequently occurs in the
season when these fish are caught and shipped to the market. In Hokkaido, the
occurrence is high in winter, especially November to March when the cod are
caught in large numbers and in August when halibut are cheap [16, 17].

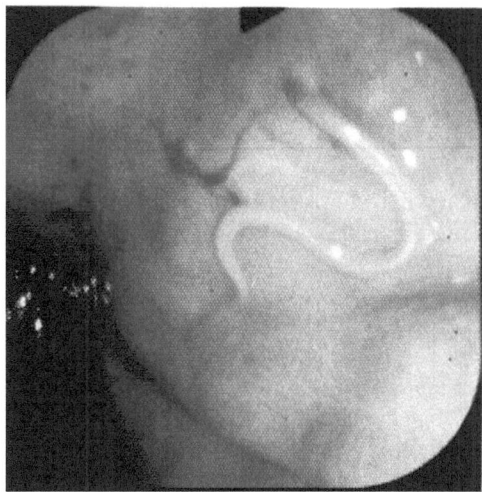

Fig. 1. Endoscopic image revealing the edematous, bleeding mucosa and the living, penetrating *Pseudoterranova decipiens* larva at the lesser curvature of the gastric body. Endoscopically, it is easy to differentiate *Pseudoterranova decipiens* from *Anisakis simplex* larvae, because the former are yellowish-brown and bigger than the latter

Sites of Penetration in Stomach

While *Anisakis simplex* larvae normally penetrate all parts of the stomach, showing no particularly dominant site, *Pseudoterranova decipiens* larvae usually penetrate the body of the stomach or the major curvature side of the cardia [14, 16, 17]. In view of the fact that rabbits orally administered with live *Pseudoterranova decipiens* larvae show no dominant site, the possibility exists that if the number of cases increases, the situation will become the same as with *Anisakis simplex* larvae [16, 17].

Endoscopic Findings

Acute gastric mucosal lesions caused by the penetration of the larvae present similar findings regardless of the kind of larva [9, 14, 15]. Mucosal lesions of gastric terranovasis can be classified according to the major endoscopic findings as follows: mucosal redness in 25% of cases, mucosal swelling with redness 34.3%, bleeding 9.3%, erosion formation 21.4%, and virtually no mucosal finding 10% [9]. Biopsy from the sites of penetration show subepithelial edema, fibrination, cellular (noneosinophilic) infiltration, and proliferation of lymph follicles but no eosinophilic phlegmon. Only changes common in already known nonspecific gastritis or virtually normal features of the mucosa are noted [6]. It is fairly easy on endoscopic observation of the penetrating larva to distinguish between *Anisakis simplex* and *Pseudoterranova decipiens* larvae (Fig. 1) [9, 14, 15]. The former is short, fine, white, and threadlike, while the latter is longer, thicker, yellowish-brown, and stringlike. Thus, *Pseudoterranova decipiens* larvae are longer than *Anisakis simplex* larvae such that endoscopic diagnosis is relatively easy.

Immunological Findings

Suzuki and Oishi [4] and Asaishi et al. [18] sensitized rabbits by intraperitoneal administration of *Anisakis simplex* larvae and by oral administration of eggs, including larvae of *Ascaris lumbricoides suum* and *Toxocara canis*. Into the gastric walls of the sensitized rabbits, they then injected body extracts of *Anisakis simplex* larvae, *Pseudoterranova decipiens* larvae, and adults of *Ascaris lumbricoides suum* and *Toxocara canis*, which had been made water-insoluble after chemical combination with cyanogen bromide-activated Sepharose 4B. The histological reactions were compared after 24 h. Strong edematous reaction with eosinophilic infiltration was noted at the sites where the extract antigen injected was of the same kind of larva used in sensitization, but the reaction was slight at the sites where an antigen of a different combination was given. Interestingly, the reaction to *Pseudoterranova decipiens* larval extract antigen in rabbits sensitized by *Anisakis simplex* larvae was almost the same as that to *Anisakis simplex* larval extract antigen. Moreover, in a Magnum apparatus, the authors set up pieces of a guinea pig ileum orally sensitized by *Anisakis simplex* larvae and eggs, including larvae of *Ascaris lumbricoides suum* and *Toxocara canis*, and dipped them into the body extract solutions of *Anisakis simplex* and *Pseudoterranova decipiens* larvae and adults of *Ascaris lumbricoides suum* and *Toxocara canis* [4, 19]. A strong reaction occurred in the homologous combination, with pronounced tetanic contraction of the piece of ileum as compared with a slight reaction in the heterologous combination. In this experiment, it was also noted that the piece of ileum sensitized by *Anisakis simplex* larva exhibited the same degree of reaction to *Pseudoterranova decipiens* larval extract solution as to *Anisakis simplex* larval extract solution. Furthermore, Suzuki and Oishi [4] extracted characteristic hemoglobin from the perienteric fluid of *Anisakis simplex* larvae and by means of desk electrophoresis and immunoelectrophoresis demonstrated that this hemoglobin is the antigen substance with the greatest specificity. They also found, using the fluorescent antibody method, that the somatic antigen of perienteric fluid reacts specifically only with the perienterium and deeper layers of the epidermis of *Anisakis simplex* and *Pseudoterranova decipiens* larvae, but not at all with *Contracaecum* larvae and adults of *Toxocara canis et cati* and *Ascaris lumbricoides suum* [20–22]. A series of these experimental results revealed that *Anisakis simplex* and *Pseudoterranova decipiens* larvae share common antigens, suggesting that severe gastric symptoms due to *Pseudoterranova decipiens* larvae can arise from a cross reaction in the human body already sensitized by *Anisakis simplex* larvae or vice versa [4].

In addition, excellent immunological studies have been carried out, including latex agglutination reactions produced on paired sera [23] and the production of monoclonal antibodies to *Anisakis simplex* larvae [24]. All these have been achieved mainly with *Anisakis simplex* larvae. Studies on *Pseudoterranova decipiens* larvae remain to be done. But, with the complete elucidation of the antigen structures of *Anisakis simplex* larvae expected in the near future, the immunological anslysis of *Pseudoterranova decipiens* larvae is expected to make remarkable progress.

Summary

At present, the only parasitic site of *Pseudoterranova decipiens* larvae in the human body is the stomach; it is found in a fulminant form, showing acute symptoms.

In Japan, gastric terranovasis is found frequently in the northern region (especially Hokkaido); in the southern regions (especially the Kyushu region), it occurs very rarely or not at all. In Hokkaido, where gastric anisakiasis is most frequent, anisakiasis and terranvasis occur in a ratio of 2:1, respectively. This difference may be explained by the fact that the parasitization of sea fish by *Pseudoterranova decipiens* larvae is limited to a few northern sea fish, such as cod and halibut.

Anisakis simplex and *Pseudoterranova decipiens* larvae do not cause essentially different lesions to acute gastric mucosal lesions caused by other *Anisakidae* larvae. With regard to the months of the year when infection commonly occurs, however, there is a difference in the frequency according to the season when the fish parasitized by *Anisakidae* larvae commonly appear on the market. At such times, the pentrating site in the human stomach differs somewhat between the two larval types.

Both larvae cause identical endoscopic findings in the human gastric mucosa. Endoscopic differential diagnosis of the penetrating larvae is easy. On endoscopic observation, *Anisakis simplex* larvae are short, fine, white, and threadlike, while *Pseudoterranova decipiens* larvae have a longer, thicker, yellowish-brown, and stringlike appearance.

The presence of an antigen common to both *Anisakis simplex* and *Pseudoterranova decipiens* larvae suggests that cross reactions are involved in bringing about gastric anisakiasis.

Since understanding of the structure of the *Anisakis simplex* larva antigen is at an advanced stage, it is expected that the immunological analysis of *Pseudoterranova decipiens* larvae will be further established in the near future.

References

1. Kagei N, Yanagawa I, Nagano K, Oishi K (1972) A larva of *Terranova* sp. causing acute abdominal syndrome in a woman. Jpn J Parasitol 21: 262–265
2. Nagano K, Takagi K, Yanagawa I, Oishi K, Kagei N (1973) Acute heterocheilidiasis of the stomach (due to *Terranova decipiens*). Stomach Intestine 8: 81–85
3. Suzuki H, Ohnuma H, Krasawa Y, Ohbayashi M, Koyama T, Kumada M, Yokogawa M (1972) *Terranova* (Nematoda; *Anisakidae*) infection in man: I. Clinical features of five cases of *Terranova* larva infection. Jpn J Parasitol 21: 252–256
4. Suzuki M, Oishi K (1974) Parasites on Alaska pollacks: VII. Larval penetration test against agar-gel. Fishes and *Anisakis* (No. 7 Fisheries scientific series). Japanese Society of Scientific Fisheries. Kohseishakohseikaku, Tokyo, pp 123–125 (in Japanese)

5. Oishi K (1974) Experimental studies of larval per oral infection (*Terranova* and *Contracaecum* larvae) on rabbits. In: Proceedings of Spring Congress of Japanese Society of Scientific Fisheries, April 1974, Tokyo, p 175 (in Japanese)

6. Nagano K, Sasaki Y, Ohtani N, Tokutomi Y, Nakaya S, Oishi K (1976) On biopsy of acute heterocheilidiasis of the stomach. Stomach Intestine 11: 195–201

7. Suzuki T, Ihikura H (1974) Pathogenic mechanisms, symptoms and diagnosis of anisakiasis. Fishes and *Anisakis*, (No. 7 Fisheries Scientific Series). Japanese Society of Scientific Fisheries. Kohseishakokseikaku, Tokyo, pp 58–72 (in Japanese)

8. Koyama T, Araki J, Machida M, Karasawa Y (1982) Current problems on anisakiasis. Modern Media 28: 434–443 (in Japanese)

9. Nagano K (1984) The individual review of the heterocheilidiasis (as a synonym for the anisakiasis). J Med Ass South Hokkaido 20: 302–312 (in Japanese)

10. Kagei N (1974) List of fishes infected *Anisakidae* larvae. Fishes and *Anisakis* (No. 7 Fisheries scientific series). Japanese Society of Scientific Fisheries. Kohseisyakohseikaku, Tokyo, pp 98–107 (in Japanese)

11. Namiki M, Morsoka T, Kawauchi H, Ueda N, Sekiya C, Nakagawa K, Furuta T, Ohguro T, Kamada H (1970) Diagnosis of acute gastric anisakiasis. Stomach Intestine 5: 1437–1440 (in Japanese)

12. Swada Y, Moriyama Y, Ebina T, Sasaki H, Yoshida Y, Tanabe K, Chiba R (1983) Gastric terranovasis: Report of 14 cases. Gastroenterol Endosc 25: 713–717

13. Sato J, Sudo T, Takemoto T, Kimura M, Yonekawa M, Yonekawa A (1984) Clinical studies of acute gastric anisakiasis (15 cases), especially anisakiasis caused by *Terranova* larva type A. Gastroenterol Endosc 26: 2137 (in Japanese)

14. Nagano K (1974) Gastric heterocheilidiasis. J Med Ass South Hokkaido 10: 58–63 (in Japanese)

15. Doi K (1973) Clinical aspects of acute heterocheilidiasis of the stomach (due to larvae of *Anisakis* and *Terranova decipiens*). Stomach Intestine 8: 1513–1518

16. Nagano K (1974) Acute gastric symptoms by *Terranova* larvae. Fishes and *Anisakis* (No. 7 Fisheries Scientific Series). Japanese Society of Scientific Fisheries Kohseishakokseikaku, Tokyo, pp 73–85 (in Japanese)

17. Nagano K, Sasaki Y, Otani N, Ebisawa K, Oishi K, Tokutomi Y, Nakaya S (1975) Investigation of acute gastric heterocheilidiasis, especially gastric terranovasis. Int Med 36: 1030–1037 (in Japanese)

18. Asaishi K, Suzuki T, Sato Y, Kenmotsu M, Otsuru M (1974) Studies on pathogenic mechanisms of anisakiasis: II. Histologic changes of stomach wall due to the injection of worm extracts. Jpn J Parasitol 23: 34 (in Japanese)

19. Sato Y, Suzuki T, Yamashita T, Otsuru M (1974) Studies on pathogenic mechanisms of anisakiasis: I. Anaphylactic reactions of segmented guinea-pig intestine. Jpn J Parasitol 23: 74 (in Japanese)

20. Asaishi K, Ishikura H, Hyasaka H, Shiraki T, Suzuki T, Otsuru M (1970) Experiments for the application of fluorescent antibody method to histological diagnosis of anisakiasis: II. Jpn J Parasitol 19: 341 (in Japanese)

21. Shiraki T, Suzuki T, Otsuru M, Asaishi K (1971) Experiments for the application of fluorescent anitbody method to histological diagnosis of anisakiasis: III. Jpn J Parasitol 20: 16 (in Japanese)

22. Shiraki T, Suzuki T, Otsuru M, Sato Y, Kenmotsu M (1973) Experiments for the application of fluorescent antibody method to histological diagnosis of anisakiasis: II. Antigenic analysis of *Anisakis* larva, especially on the cuticular antigen. Jpn J Parasitol 22: 141–145

23. Yoshimura H (1984) Gastric anisakiasis in the Kanazawa district and latex agglutination. Gastroenterol Endosc 26: 2134 (in Japanese)

24. Takahashi S, Hayasaka H, Ishikura H, Koshida H, Kikuchi H (1985) Attempts to generate monoclonal antibodies against *Anisakis* larvae. In: Ishikura H (ed) Anisakiasis (Supplementation no. 6, 1984–1985). Ishikura Hospital, Iwanai, p 7 (in Japanese)

Subject Index